Women's Health Care Nurse Practitioner Exam
Part 1 of 2

SECRETS

Study Guide
Your Key to Exam Success

NP Test Review for the
Nurse Practitioner Exam

Dear Future Exam Success Story:

First of all, **THANK YOU** for purchasing Mometrix study materials!

Second, congratulations! You are one of the few determined test-takers who are committed to doing whatever it takes to excel on your exam. **You have come to the right place.** We developed these study materials with one goal in mind: to deliver you the information you need in a format that's concise and easy to use.

In addition to optimizing your guide for the content of the test, we've outlined our recommended steps for breaking down the preparation process into small, attainable goals so you can make sure you stay on track.

We've also analyzed the entire test-taking process, identifying the most common pitfalls and showing how you can overcome them and be ready for any curveball the test throws you.

Standardized testing is one of the biggest obstacles on your road to success, which only increases the importance of doing well in the high-pressure, high-stakes environment of test day. Your results on this test could have a significant impact on your future, and this guide provides the information and practical advice to help you achieve your full potential on test day.

Your success is our success

We would love to hear from you! If you would like to share the story of your exam success or if you have any questions or comments in regard to our products, please contact us at **800-673-8175** or **support@mometrix.com**.

Thanks again for your business and we wish you continued success!

Sincerely,
The Mometrix Test Preparation Team

Need more help? Check out our flashcards at: http://MometrixFlashcards.com/NP

TABLE OF CONTENTS

Introduction

Thank you for purchasing this resource! You have made the choice to prepare yourself for a test that could have a huge impact on your future, and this guide is designed to help you be fully ready for test day. Obviously, it's important to have a solid understanding of the test material, but you also need to be prepared for the unique environment and stressors of the test, so that you can perform to the best of your abilities.

For this purpose, the first section that appears in this guide is the **Secret Keys**. We've devoted countless hours to meticulously researching what works and what doesn't, and we've boiled down our findings to the five most impactful steps you can take to improve your performance on the test. We start at the beginning with study planning and move through the preparation process, all the way to the testing strategies that will help you get the most out of what you know when you're finally sitting in front of the test.

We recommend that you start preparing for your test as far in advance as possible. However, if you've bought this guide as a last-minute study resource and only have a few days before your test, we recommend that you skip over the first two Secret Keys since they address a long-term study plan.

If you struggle with **test anxiety**, we strongly encourage you to check out our recommendations for how you can overcome it. Test anxiety is a formidable foe, but it can be beaten, and we want to make sure you have the tools you need to defeat it.

Secret Key #1 – Plan Big, Study Small

There's a lot riding on your performance. If you want to ace this test, you're going to need to keep your skills sharp and the material fresh in your mind. You need a plan that lets you review everything you need to know while still fitting in your schedule. We'll break this strategy down into three categories.

Information Organization

Start with the information you already have: the official test outline. From this, you can make a complete list of all the concepts you need to cover before the test. Organize these concepts into groups that can be studied together, and create a list of any related vocabulary you need to learn so you can brush up on any difficult terms. You'll want to keep this vocabulary list handy once you actually start studying since you may need to add to it along the way.

Time Management

Once you have your set of study concepts, decide how to spread them out over the time you have left before the test. Break your study plan into small, clear goals so you have a manageable task for each day and know exactly what you're doing. Then just focus on one small step at a time. When you manage your time this way, you don't need to spend hours at a time studying. Studying a small block of content for a short period each day helps you retain information better and avoid stressing over how much you have left to do. You can relax knowing that you have a plan to cover everything in time. In order for this strategy to be effective though, you have to start studying early and stick to your schedule. Avoid the exhaustion and futility that comes from last-minute cramming!

Study Environment

The environment you study in has a big impact on your learning. Studying in a coffee shop, while probably more enjoyable, is not likely to be as fruitful as studying in a quiet room. It's important to keep distractions to a minimum. You're only planning to study for a short block of time, so make the most of it. Don't pause to check your phone or get up to find a snack. It's also important to **avoid multitasking**. Research has consistently shown that multitasking will make your studying dramatically less effective. Your study area should also be comfortable and well-lit so you don't have the distraction of straining your eyes or sitting on an uncomfortable chair.

The time of day you study is also important. You want to be rested and alert. Don't wait until just before bedtime. Study when you'll be most likely to comprehend and remember. Even better, if you know what time of day your test will be, set that time aside for study. That way your brain will be used to working on that subject at that specific time and you'll have a better chance of recalling information.

Finally, it can be helpful to team up with others who are studying for the same test. Your actual studying should be done in as isolated an environment as possible, but the work of organizing the information and setting up the study plan can be divided up. In between study sessions, you can discuss with your teammates the concepts that you're all studying and quiz each other on the details. Just be sure that your teammates are as serious about the test as you are. If you find that your study time is being replaced with social time, you might need to find a new team.

Secret Key #2 – Make Your Studying Count

You're devoting a lot of time and effort to preparing for this test, so you want to be absolutely certain it will pay off. This means doing more than just reading the content and hoping you can remember it on test day. It's important to make every minute of study count. There are two main areas you can focus on to make your studying count:

Retention

It doesn't matter how much time you study if you can't remember the material. You need to make sure you are retaining the concepts. To check your retention of the information you're learning, try recalling it at later times with minimal prompting. Try carrying around flashcards and glance at one or two from time to time or ask a friend who's also studying for the test to quiz you.

To enhance your retention, look for ways to put the information into practice so that you can apply it rather than simply recalling it. If you're using the information in practical ways, it will be much easier to remember. Similarly, it helps to solidify a concept in your mind if you're not only reading it to yourself but also explaining it to someone else. Ask a friend to let you teach them about a concept you're a little shaky on (or speak aloud to an imaginary audience if necessary). As you try to summarize, define, give examples, and answer your friend's questions, you'll understand the concepts better and they will stay with you longer. Finally, step back for a big picture view and ask yourself how each piece of information fits with the whole subject. When you link the different concepts together and see them working together as a whole, it's easier to remember the individual components.

Finally, practice showing your work on any multi-step problems, even if you're just studying. Writing out each step you take to solve a problem will help solidify the process in your mind, and you'll be more likely to remember it during the test.

Modality

Modality simply refers to the means or method by which you study. Choosing a study modality that fits your own individual learning style is crucial. No two people learn best in exactly the same way, so it's important to know your strengths and use them to your advantage.

For example, if you learn best by visualization, focus on visualizing a concept in your mind and draw an image or a diagram. Try color-coding your notes, illustrating them, or creating symbols that will trigger your mind to recall a learned concept. If you learn best by hearing or discussing information, find a study partner who learns the same way or read aloud to yourself. Think about how to put the information in your own words. Imagine that you are giving a lecture on the topic and record yourself so you can listen to it later.

For any learning style, flashcards can be helpful. Organize the information so you can take advantage of spare moments to review. Underline key words or phrases. Use different colors for different categories. Mnemonic devices (such as creating a short list in which every item starts with the same letter) can also help with retention. Find what works best for you and use it to store the information in your mind most effectively and easily.

Secret Key #3 – Practice the Right Way

Your success on test day depends not only on how many hours you put into preparing, but also on whether you prepared the right way. It's good to check along the way to see if your studying is paying off. One of the most effective ways to do this is by taking practice tests to evaluate your progress. Practice tests are useful because they show exactly where you need to improve. Every time you take a practice test, pay special attention to these three groups of questions:

- The questions you got wrong
- The questions you had to guess on, even if you guessed right
- The questions you found difficult or slow to work through

This will show you exactly what your weak areas are, and where you need to devote more study time. Ask yourself why each of these questions gave you trouble. Was it because you didn't understand the material? Was it because you didn't remember the vocabulary? Do you need more repetitions on this type of question to build speed and confidence? Dig into those questions and figure out how you can strengthen your weak areas as you go back to review the material.

Additionally, many practice tests have a section explaining the answer choices. It can be tempting to read the explanation and think that you now have a good understanding of the concept. However, an explanation likely only covers part of the question's broader context. Even if the explanation makes sense, **go back and investigate** every concept related to the question until you're positive you have a thorough understanding.

As you go along, keep in mind that the practice test is just that: practice. Memorizing these questions and answers will not be very helpful on the actual test because it is unlikely to have any of the same exact questions. If you only know the right answers to the sample questions, you won't be prepared for the real thing. **Study the concepts** until you understand them fully, and then you'll be able to answer any question that shows up on the test.

It's important to wait on the practice tests until you're ready. If you take a test on your first day of study, you may be overwhelmed by the amount of material covered and how much you need to learn. Work up to it gradually.

On test day, you'll need to be prepared for answering questions, managing your time, and using the test-taking strategies you've learned. It's a lot to balance, like a mental marathon that will have a big impact on your future. Like training for a marathon, you'll need to start slowly and work your way up. When test day arrives, you'll be ready.

Start with the strategies you've read in the first two Secret Keys—plan your course and study in the way that works best for you. If you have time, consider using multiple study resources to get different approaches to the same concepts. It can be helpful to see difficult concepts from more than one angle. Then find a good source for practice tests. Many times, the test website will suggest potential study resources or provide sample tests.

Practice Test Strategy

If you're able to find at least three practice tests, we recommend this strategy:

1. Take the first test with no time constraints and with your notes and study guide handy. Take your time and focus on applying the strategies you've learned.
2. Take the second practice test open-book as well, but set a timer and practice pacing yourself to finish in time.
3. Take any other practice tests as if it were test day. Set a timer and put away your study materials. Sit at a table or desk in a quiet room, imagine yourself at the testing center, and answer questions as quickly and accurately as possible.
4. Keep repeating step 3 on a regular basis until you run out of practice tests or it's time for the actual test. Your mind will be ready for the schedule and stress of test day, and you'll be able to focus on recalling the material you've learned.

Secret Key #4 – Pace Yourself

Once you're fully prepared for the material on the test, your biggest challenge on test day will be managing your time. Just knowing that the clock is ticking can make you panic even if you have plenty of time left. Work on pacing yourself so you can build confidence against the time constraints of the exam. Pacing is a difficult skill to master, especially in a high-pressure environment, so **practice is vital**.

Set time expectations for your pace based on how much time is available. For example, if a section has 60 questions and the time limit is 30 minutes, you know you have to average 30 seconds or less per question in order to answer them all. Although 30 seconds is the hard limit, set 25 seconds per question as your goal, so you reserve extra time to spend on harder questions. When you budget extra time for the harder questions, you no longer have any reason to stress when those questions take longer to answer.

Don't let this time expectation distract you from working through the test at a calm, steady pace, but keep it in mind so you don't spend too much time on any one question. Recognize that taking extra time on one question you don't understand may keep you from answering two that you do understand later in the test. If your time limit for a question is up and you're still not sure of the answer, mark it and move on, and come back to it later if the time and the test format allow. If the testing format doesn't allow you to return to earlier questions, just make an educated guess; then put it out of your mind and move on.

On the easier questions, be careful not to rush. It may seem wise to hurry through them so you have more time for the challenging ones, but it's not worth missing one if you know the concept and just didn't take the time to read the question fully. Work efficiently but make sure you understand the question and have looked at all of the answer choices, since more than one may seem right at first.

Even if you're paying attention to the time, you may find yourself a little behind at some point. You should speed up to get back on track, but do so wisely. Don't panic; just take a few seconds less on each question until you're caught up. Don't guess without thinking, but do look through the answer choices and eliminate any you know are wrong. If you can get down to two choices, it is often worthwhile to guess from those. Once you've chosen an answer, move on and don't dwell on any that you skipped or had to hurry through. If a question was taking too long, chances are it was one of the harder ones, so you weren't as likely to get it right anyway.

On the other hand, if you find yourself getting ahead of schedule, it may be beneficial to slow down a little. The more quickly you work, the more likely you are to make a careless mistake that will affect your score. You've budgeted time for each question, so don't be afraid to spend that time. Practice an efficient but careful pace to get the most out of the time you have.

Secret Key #5 – Have a Plan for Guessing

When you're taking the test, you may find yourself stuck on a question. Some of the answer choices seem better than others, but you don't see the one answer choice that is obviously correct. What do you do?

The scenario described above is very common, yet most test takers have not effectively prepared for it. Developing and practicing a plan for guessing may be one of the single most effective uses of your time as you get ready for the exam.

In developing your plan for guessing, there are three questions to address:

- When should you start the guessing process?
- How should you narrow down the choices?
- Which answer should you choose?

When to Start the Guessing Process

Unless your plan for guessing is to select C every time (which, despite its merits, is not what we recommend), you need to leave yourself enough time to apply your answer elimination strategies. Since you have a limited amount of time for each question, that means that if you're going to give yourself the best shot at guessing correctly, you have to decide quickly whether or not you will guess.

Of course, the best-case scenario is that you don't have to guess at all, so first, see if you can answer the question based on your knowledge of the subject and basic reasoning skills. Focus on the key words in the question and try to jog your memory of related topics. Give yourself a chance to bring the knowledge to mind, but once you realize that you don't have (or you can't access) the knowledge you need to answer the question, it's time to start the guessing process.

It's almost always better to start the guessing process too early than too late. It only takes a few seconds to remember something and answer the question from knowledge. Carefully eliminating wrong answer choices takes longer. Plus, going through the process of eliminating answer choices can actually help jog your memory.

Summary: Start the guessing process as soon as you decide that you can't answer the question based on your knowledge.

How to Narrow Down the Choices

The next chapter in this book (**Test-Taking Strategies**) includes a wide range of strategies for how to approach questions and how to look for answer choices to eliminate. You will definitely want to read those carefully, practice them, and figure out which ones work best for you. Here though, we're going to address a mindset rather than a particular strategy.

Your chances of guessing an answer correctly depend on how many options you are choosing from.

How many choices you have	How likely you are to guess correctly
5	20%
4	25%
3	33%
2	50%
1	100%

You can see from this chart just how valuable it is to be able to eliminate incorrect answers and make an educated guess, but there are two things that many test takers do that cause them to miss out on the benefits of guessing:

- Accidentally eliminating the correct answer
- Selecting an answer based on an impression

We'll look at the first one here, and the second one in the next section.

To avoid accidentally eliminating the correct answer, we recommend a thought exercise called **the $5 challenge**. In this challenge, you only eliminate an answer choice from contention if you are willing to bet $5 on it being wrong. Why $5? Five dollars is a small but not insignificant amount of money. It's an amount you could afford to lose but wouldn't want to throw away. And while losing $5 once might not hurt too much, doing it twenty times will set you back $100. In the same way, each small decision you make—eliminating a choice here, guessing on a question there—won't by itself impact your score very much, but when you put them all together, they can make a big difference. By holding each answer choice elimination decision to a higher standard, you can reduce the risk of accidentally eliminating the correct answer.

The $5 challenge can also be applied in a positive sense: If you are willing to bet $5 that an answer choice *is* correct, go ahead and mark it as correct.

Summary: Only eliminate an answer choice if you are willing to bet $5 that it is wrong.

Which Answer to Choose

You're taking the test. You've run into a hard question and decided you'll have to guess. You've eliminated all the answer choices you're willing to bet $5 on. Now you have to pick an answer. Why do we even need to talk about this? Why can't you just pick whichever one you feel like when the time comes?

The answer to these questions is that if you don't come into the test with a plan, you'll rely on your impression to select an answer choice, and if you do that, you risk falling into a trap. The test writers know that everyone who takes their test will be guessing on some of the questions, so they intentionally write wrong answer choices to seem plausible. You still have to pick an answer though, and if the wrong answer choices are designed to look right, how can you ever be sure that you're not falling for their trap? The best solution we've found to this dilemma is to take the decision out of your hands entirely. Here is the process we recommend:

Once you've eliminated any choices that you are confident (willing to bet $5) are wrong, select the first remaining choice as your answer.

Whether you choose to select the first remaining choice, the second, or the last, the important thing is that you use some preselected standard. Using this approach guarantees that you will not be enticed into selecting an answer choice that looks right, because you are not basing your decision on how the answer choices look.

This is not meant to make you question your knowledge. Instead, it is to help you recognize the difference between your knowledge and your impressions. There's a huge difference between thinking an answer is right because of what you know, and thinking an answer is right because it looks or sounds like it should be right.

Summary: To ensure that your selection is appropriately random, make a predetermined selection from among all answer choices you have not eliminated.

Test-Taking Strategies

This section contains a list of test-taking strategies that you may find helpful as you work through the test. By taking what you know and applying logical thought, you can maximize your chances of answering any question correctly!

It is very important to realize that every question is different and every person is different: no single strategy will work on every question, and no single strategy will work for every person. That's why we've included all of them here, so you can try them out and determine which ones work best for different types of questions and which ones work best for you.

Question Strategies

Read Carefully

Read the question and answer choices carefully. Don't miss the question because you misread the terms. You have plenty of time to read each question thoroughly and make sure you understand what is being asked. Yet a happy medium must be attained, so don't waste too much time. You must read carefully, but efficiently.

Contextual Clues

Look for contextual clues. If the question includes a word you are not familiar with, look at the immediate context for some indication of what the word might mean. Contextual clues can often give you all the information you need to decipher the meaning of an unfamiliar word. Even if you can't determine the meaning, you may be able to narrow down the possibilities enough to make a solid guess at the answer to the question.

Prefixes

If you're having trouble with a word in the question or answer choices, try dissecting it. Take advantage of every clue that the word might include. Prefixes and suffixes can be a huge help. Usually they allow you to determine a basic meaning. Pre- means before, post- means after, pro - is positive, de- is negative. From prefixes and suffixes, you can get an idea of the general meaning of the word and try to put it into context.

Hedge Words

Watch out for critical hedge words, such as *likely*, *may*, *can*, *sometimes*, *often*, *almost*, *mostly*, *usually*, *generally*, *rarely*, and *sometimes*. Question writers insert these hedge phrases to cover every possibility. Often an answer choice will be wrong simply because it leaves no room for exception. Be on guard for answer choices that have definitive words such as *exactly* and *always*.

Switchback Words

Stay alert for *switchbacks*. These are the words and phrases frequently used to alert you to shifts in thought. The most common switchback words are *but*, *although*, and *however*. Others include *nevertheless, on the other hand, even though, while, in spite of, despite, regardless of*. Switchback words are important to catch because they can change the direction of the question or an answer choice.

- 10 -

Face Value

When in doubt, use common sense. Accept the situation in the problem at face value. Don't read too much into it. These problems will not require you to make wild assumptions. If you have to go beyond creativity and warp time or space in order to have an answer choice fit the question, then you should move on and consider the other answer choices. These are normal problems rooted in reality. The applicable relationship or explanation may not be readily apparent, but it is there for you to figure out. Use your common sense to interpret anything that isn't clear.

Answer Choice Strategies

Answer Selection

The most thorough way to pick an answer choice is to identify and eliminate wrong answers until only one is left, then confirm it is the correct answer. Sometimes an answer choice may immediately seem right, but be careful. The test writers will usually put more than one reasonable answer choice on each question, so take a second to read all of them and make sure that the other choices are not equally obvious. As long as you have time left, it is better to read every answer choice than to pick the first one that looks right without checking the others.

Answer Choice Families

An answer choice family consists of two (in rare cases, three) answer choices that are very similar in construction and cannot all be true at the same time. If you see two answer choices that are direct opposites or parallels, one of them is usually the correct answer. For instance, if one answer choice says that quantity x increases and another either says that quantity x decreases (opposite) or says that quantity y increases (parallel), then those answer choices would fall into the same family. An answer choice that doesn't match the construction of the answer choice family is more likely to be incorrect. Most questions will not have answer choice families, but when they do appear, you should be prepared to recognize them.

Eliminate Answers

Eliminate answer choices as soon as you realize they are wrong, but make sure you consider all possibilities. If you are eliminating answer choices and realize that the last one you are left with is also wrong, don't panic. Start over and consider each choice again. There may be something you missed the first time that you will realize on the second pass.

Avoid Fact Traps

Don't be distracted by an answer choice that is factually true but doesn't answer the question. You are looking for the choice that answers the question. Stay focused on what the question is asking for so you don't accidentally pick an answer that is true but incorrect. Always go back to the question and make sure the answer choice you've selected actually answers the question and is not merely a true statement.

Extreme Statements

In general, you should avoid answers that put forth extreme actions as standard practice or proclaim controversial ideas as established fact. An answer choice that states the "process should be used in certain situations, if..." is much more likely to be correct than one that states the "process should be discontinued completely." The first is a calm rational statement and doesn't even make a definitive, uncompromising stance, using a hedge word *if* to provide wiggle room, whereas the second choice is a radical idea and far more extreme.

Benchmark

As you read through the answer choices and you come across one that seems to answer the question well, mentally select that answer choice. This is not your final answer, but it's the one that will help you evaluate the other answer choices. The one that you selected is your benchmark or standard for judging each of the other answer choices. Every other answer choice must be compared to your benchmark. That choice is correct until proven otherwise by another answer choice beating it. If you find a better answer, then that one becomes your new benchmark. Once you've decided that no other choice answers the question as well as your benchmark, you have your final answer.

Predict the Answer

Before you even start looking at the answer choices, it is often best to try to predict the answer. When you come up with the answer on your own, it is easier to avoid distractions and traps because you will know exactly what to look for. The right answer choice is unlikely to be word-for-word what you came up with, but it should be a close match. Even if you are confident that you have the right answer, you should still take the time to read each option before moving on.

General Strategies

Tough Questions

If you are stumped on a problem or it appears too hard or too difficult, don't waste time. Move on! Remember though, if you can quickly check for obviously incorrect answer choices, your chances of guessing correctly are greatly improved. Before you completely give up, at least try to knock out a couple of possible answers. Eliminate what you can and then guess at the remaining answer choices before moving on.

Check Your Work

Since you will probably not know every term listed and the answer to every question, it is important that you get credit for the ones that you do know. Don't miss any questions through careless mistakes. If at all possible, try to take a second to look back over your answer selection and make sure you've selected the correct answer choice and haven't made a costly careless mistake (such as marking an answer choice that you didn't mean to mark). This quick double check should more than pay for itself in caught mistakes for the time it costs.

Pace Yourself

It's easy to be overwhelmed when you're looking at a page full of questions; your mind is confused and full of random thoughts, and the clock is ticking down faster than you would like. Calm down and maintain the pace that you have set for yourself. Especially as you get down to the last few minutes of the test, don't let the small numbers on the clock make you panic. As long as you are on track by monitoring your pace, you are guaranteed to have time for each question.

Don't Rush

It is very easy to make errors when you are in a hurry. Maintaining a fast pace in answering questions is pointless if it makes you miss questions that you would have gotten right otherwise. Test writers like to include distracting information and wrong answers that seem right. Taking a little extra time to avoid careless mistakes can make all the difference in your test score. Find a pace that allows you to be confident in the answers that you select.

Keep Moving

Panicking will not help you pass the test, so do your best to stay calm and keep moving. Taking deep breaths and going through the answer elimination steps you practiced can help to break through a stress barrier and keep your pace.

Final Notes

The combination of a solid foundation of content knowledge and the confidence that comes from practicing your plan for applying that knowledge is the key to maximizing your performance on test day. As your foundation of content knowledge is built up and strengthened, you'll find that the strategies included in this chapter become more and more effective in helping you quickly sift through the distractions and traps of the test to isolate the correct answer.

Now it's time to move on to the test content chapters of this book, but be sure to keep your goal in mind. As you read, think about how you will be able to apply this information on the test. If you've already seen sample questions for the test and you have an idea of the question format and style, try to come up with questions of your own that you can answer based on what you're reading. This will give you valuable practice applying your knowledge in the same ways you can expect to on test day.

Good luck and good studying!

Physical Assessment and Diagnostic Evaluation

Health history

The main components of the health history are as follows:

- The reason for today's visit
- The patient's description of the illness or injury for which she is seeking attention
- Past medical history (PMH): childhood and adult diseases or injuries, history of abuse or rape, mental health problems, surgeries and hospitalizations, blood transfusions
- State of general health at present: tobacco or alcohol use; medications (prescription and over-the-counter [OTC]); allergies to medications, foods, animals, insect bites or stings, and other environmental factors; recent significant weight changes; immunization status; exercise pattern; home or occupational exposure to environmental hazards; and physical or mental health disabilities
- Pertinent family history: genetic or familial disease patterns
- Obstetrical history: number of pregnancies (including live births) and abortions (including miscarriages)
- Gynecological history: history of sexual activity, current sexual history, history of sexually transmitted diseases (STDs), contraceptive use
- Desire for children
- Review of systems (ROS)

SOAP format

The following describes the SOAP format for recording information in the patient's medical chart and the information that should be recorded under each heading:

- **S** - Subjective information: all components of the health history
- **O** - Objective information: physical examination findings (including pertinent positives and negatives), laboratory tests ordered and their results, procedures ordered and their results
- **A** - Assessment: differential diagnosis and a ranking of the likelihood of each diagnosis; rationale for each diagnosis; a statement of whether each diagnosis is ruled in or ruled out
- **P** - Plan: plan of action based on the information presented under the previous headings; information about further tests to be ordered, referrals to specialists, and follow-up visit

History of chief complaint

Adults often present with a myriad of health problems, so a problem-based assessment, focusing on finding a solution to chief complaints and current health problems, can be effective. Problem-based assessment requires a thorough history to create a problem list. This approach does not preclude a complete exam, which might identify problems that the patient has neglected, but the focus remains on the problem list generated. The list should be prioritized to ensure that the most critical issues (blood in the stool) are thoroughly assessed before less critical issues (occasional insomnia). Once a problem is identified, then differential diagnoses are determined. With adults, there may be a combination of physical and psychosocial elements to a problem. For example, urinary problems may relate to dehydration, lack of mobility, poor hygiene, medications, or disease. Appropriate diagnostic tests, further assessments, and interventions are completed as needed to diagnose and resolve problems.

Systems review

The elements of a systems review are as follows:

- **General** - Note normal weight, changes in weight, sleeping patterns, malaise, weakness, fever.
- **Head:**
  - Frequency or occurrence of headaches, head injuries.
  - Frequency of upper respiratory infections, nasal stuffiness, discharge, itching, hay fever, sinus congestion, and nosebleeds.
  - Condition of teeth and gums, last dental exam, hoarseness, bleeding gums, sore tongue, and frequency of sore throats.
- **Neck** - Swollen lymph nodes, stiffness, and goiter.
- **Eyes** - Vision (contact lenses, glasses), redness, tearing, visual disturbances, glaucoma, cataracts, and macular degeneration.
- **Ears** - Hearing, vertigo, tinnitus, earaches, and discharge.
- **Skin** - Rashes, texture changes, jaundice, nevi, dryness, and lesions.
- **Breasts** - Masses, nipple discharge, changes in nipple, date of last mammogram, and frequency of self breast exam.
- **Cardiac** - Heart problems, hypertension, heart murmurs, chest pain, paroxysmal nocturnal dyspnea, and prior ECGs or heart tests.
- **Respiratory** - Cough, sputum, dyspnea, hemoptysis, bronchitis, COPD, asthma, tuberculosis, pleurisy, and last chest x-ray and/or PPD.
- **Gastrointestinal** - Dysphagia, heartburn, appetite, nausea, vomiting, regurgitation, indigestions, frequency and character of stools, abdominal pain, food allergies/intolerances, flatus, jaundice, and hepatitis, liver, or gallbladder problems.
- **Urinary** - Frequency, nocturia, polyuria, pain or burning, hematuria, urgency, incontinence, changes in urinary stream, urinary infections, and calculi.
- **Peripheral/ Vascular** - Leg pain, cramping, varicose veins, and phlebitis.
- **Gynecologic** - Age at menarche/menopause, regularity, frequency, and duration of menses, bleeding between periods/after intercourse, discharge, premenstrual tension, postmenopausal symptoms, itching, masses, gravida/para/abortus, contraception, and sexual problems.
- **Neurologic** - Fainting, seizures, blackouts, paresis/paralysis, change in sensation (numbness, tingling), tremors, and involuntary movement.
- **Hematologic** - Bruising, bleeding, anemia, and past transfusions/reactions.
- **Endocrine** - Thyroid disease, heat/cold intolerance, diabetes, polyuria/polydipsia, excessive hunger, and excessive perspiration.
- **Psychiatric** - Mood/anxiety disorders, nervousness, tension, cognitive impairment.
- **Musculoskeletal** - Pains, stiffness, arthritis, gout, backaches, inflammatory changes, and limitations in mobility

Family history

The following are questions that can be used to elicit a patient's family history and the reasons for asking those questions:

- Number and ages of siblings: the patient's placement in the order of birth may affect the patient's mental health makeup.
- General health of the patient's siblings and parents: this information could indicate familial or genetic predispositions to diseases such as breast or ovarian cancer.
- Number and ages of children and their general health: this information can indicate familial or genetic problems. Answers about younger children's immunization status and visits to health care providers can suggest possible parental child abuse or neglect.

Sexual history

The following are questions that can be used to elicit a patient's sexual history and the reasons for asking those questions:

- Number of sexual partners during her life and within the last three months: a large number of sexual partners can not only predispose the patient to STDs but also increase the likelihood of cervical cancer. The number of partners within the last three months can suggest the likelihood of pregnancy or recently acquired STDs.
- Age at first sexual intercourse: in general, the earlier a woman becomes sexually active, the greater her likelihood of having numerous sexual partners.
- Consensual nature of first sexual intercourse: if the first sexual intercourse was nonconsensual, the patient may have emotional problems that should be addressed.
- History of sexual abuse or rape: sexual abuse or rape can predispose a patient to emotional difficulties that should be addressed by a mental health provider.

Observations before physical assessment

The following are some observations that can be made about a patient before the physical examination begins and that may suggest the patient's health status:

- The patient's speech pattern suggests her educational level and cultural background and may indicate whether she is mentally challenged or has active disease processes. For example, if she has difficulty speaking, is in obvious distress, and is holding a handkerchief in front of her mouth to catch saliva, she may have a peritonsillar abscess.
- The patient's grooming and personal hygiene habits can suggest self-esteem issues, possible substance abuse, and homelessness.
- Bearing can suggest the patient's mental status and may indicate conditions such as depression or paranoia.
- Symptoms of medical conditions such as goiter, hyperthyroidism, and skin diseases can be observed before the physical examination begins.
- "Track marks" on the forearms suggest current drug use. Track marks that have healed but have left visible scars suggest past drug use or addiction.

Physical examination

<u>Anthropometric measurements</u>

BMI

The Body Mass Index (BMI) formula uses height and weight as an indicator of obesity/malnutrition. Women often have more body fat than men. Tables are available to make calculations simple, but the BMI can be calculated manually:

$$BMI = \frac{\text{weight in lb} \times 703}{\text{height in inch}^2}$$

$$BMI = \frac{\text{weight in kilograms}}{\text{Height in meters}^2}$$

The resulting scores for adults age 20 and over are interpreted according to this chart:

Below 18.5 = Underweight
18.5 − 24.9 = Normal weight
25.0 − 29.9 = Overweight
30 and above = Obese

WHR

The Waist-to-Hip Ratio (WHR) is the ratio of fat stored about the abdomen and the fat stored around the hips. An increase in this ratio is associated with increased risk of heart disease, strokes, and diabetes. The formula:

$$WHR = \frac{\text{Waist circumference in cm}}{\text{hip circumference in cm}}$$

The waist measurement is taken at the smallest circumference, usually slightly above the umbilicus, and the hip measurement is taken at the widest part of the hips, usually about 7 in. below the waist.

The results of the calculation provide a score with risks according to gender: females >0.85/males >1 = increased risk.

TST

The Triceps skinfold thickness (TST) test evaluates fat stores, and it can be used to determine if fat is increasing while muscle mass is decreasing. The midpoint between the axilla and elbow of the nondominant arm is located, and the skin grasped at the arm edges about 1 cm above the midpoint between the thumb and index finger, moving the finger and thumb inward until a firm fold of tissue is observed. Special calipers are placed about this fold at the midpoint (right below the fingers) and squeezed for three seconds, and then a measurement taken to the nearest millimeter. The average of three measurements is used. The TST is recorded as a percentage of standard measurements, which are quantified for males and females:

Female TST = 16.5 mm
Male TST = 12.5 mm

In order to reach the percentage, the actual measurement for each test is divided by the standard measurement and that result in multiplied by 100. Thus, if the woman's TST measured 12:

$$12/16.5 = 72.7 \times 100 = 73\%$$

MAC and MAMC

The midarm circumference (MAC) measurement is obtained by measuring in centimeters at the midpoint between the axilla and elbow. MAC measures muscles, bones, and skin. The midarm muscle circumference (MAMC) is calculated by multiplying the triceps skinfold thickness (in millimeters) by pi (3.14) and subtracting the result from the midarm circumference with results in centimeters. MAMC measures lean body mass. These measurements vary considerably between individuals, so they are more useful to track muscle wasting over time than for comparisons. The MAC and MAMC are recorded as a percentage of standard measurements, which are quantified for males and females.

Female MAC = 28.5 cm
Male MAC = 29.9 cm
Female MAMC = 23.3 cm
Male MAMC = 25.3 cm

In order to reach the percentage, the actual measurement for each test is divided by the standard measurement and that result in multiplied by 100. Thus, if the MAC for a woman is 26.7:

$$26.7/28.5 = 93.6 \times 100 = 94\%$$

Vital signs

- Temperature: Body temperature should range between 36°C/96.8°F and 38°C/100.4°C. Tympanic membrane sensors provide accurate core body temperatures. Rectal temperatures are usually about 0.5°C/0.9°F higher than oral, and axillary and tympanic are about 0.5°C/0.9°F lower than oral. Use the same method for serial temperature readings.
- Pulse: Adults average from 60 to 100 bpm. Assess both apical and peripheral pulses (radial). The difference between the apical and peripheral pulse is the pulse deficit, which may indicate a weak pulse or dysrhythmia.
- Respirations: Adults average 12 to 20/min. at rest. Wait 5 to 10 min. after activity to assess respirations. Assess for 30 seconds, and multiply by 2 or for one full minute if irregularities are evident.
- Blood pressure: Optimal values <120/<80 with hypertension ≥140/≥90. Indicate patient's position (sitting, lying). Ensure cuff is positioned and fitted correctly. Wait 1 to 2 minutes before rechecking.
  - o False high readings: A cuff that is too narrow, a cuff that is too loose, arm below heart, and an unsupported arm.
  - o False low readings: A cuff that is too wide and arm above heart level.
  - o False high diastolic readings: Inflating or deflating the cuff too slowly.

Head

Examination of the head includes the following:

- Hair - Remove wigs/hairpieces. Note the quantity of hair and any pattern of loss of scalp lesions. Inspect for dandruff, nits, lesions, seborrhea (red, scaling), and sores, parting the hair.

- Shape - Note contours of skull and face, noting tenderness, enlargements, or abnormalities:
  - Cushing syndrome: Moon face, hirsutism, red cheeks.
  - Myxedema: Dry skin, hair, and eyebrows, face edematous, especially about eyes.
  - Nephrotic syndrome: Face pale and edematous, severe about eyes.
  - Parkinson's disease: Masklike facies with decreased blinking and apparent staring, usually upward as the neck flexes forward. Skin oily and patient may drool.
  - Acromegaly: Elongated head, with prominent nose, jaw, and forehead with soft-tissue enlargement.
- Nose - Note asymmetry, deformity, or signs of inflammation. Examine with otoscope:
  - Septum: Deviation, obstruction, bleeding, crusting, perforation (indication of intranasal use of cocaine and methamphetamines).
  - Mucosa: Color, exudate, edema bleeding (red and edematous with acute rhinitis and pale with allergic rhinitis).
  - Turbinates: Polyps, edema, exudate.
- Skin - Note color, pigment changes, acne, folliculitis, lesions hirsutism, and changes in texture and thickness or hair distribution.

Sinuses

Examination of the sinuses is as follows:

- Press superiorly under bony brow and on each maxillary sinus. (Tenderness with pain, fever, and nasal discharge indicates infected sinus.)
- Use transillumination in darkened room if symptoms of sinusitis: Lack of glow indicates inflammation.

Mouth

Examination of the mouth includes the mouth, gums, teeth, and gums:

- Remove dentures. Inspect lips for shape, color, dryness, and lesions and mucosa for color, pigmentation, moisture, ulcers, nodules, lesions. Note color and shape of hard palate.
- Inspect gums:
  - Gingivitis: Edema, erythema, bleeding about tooth margins.
  - Periodontitis: Edema, erythema, bleeding, pockets, receding gums.
  - Acute necrotizing gingivitis: Erythema, edema, ulcerations, and gray membranes.
  - Gingival hyperplasia: Generalized (pubertal changes, pregnancy, leukemia, phenytoin) or localized epulis (inflammatory or neoplastic).
  - Bismuth/lead line: Bluish-black discoloration 1 mm above gum margin.
  - Melanin pigmentation: Brownish discoloration (common in dark-skinned people and Addison's disease)
- Inspect teeth:
  - Caries: Chalky, to brown, to black spots in enamel.
  - Hutchinson's teeth (congenital syphilis): Small, tapered, widely spaced notched teeth.
  - Notched, abraded spots from trauma.
  - Attrition: Flattened biting surface resulting in yellow/brown stains
- Inspect the tongue:
  - Males older than 50 or heavy drinkers or smokers: Ask patient to stick tongue out, grasp with gauze, and pull to one side, examining and palpating the opposite side, then reverse (inspecting for cancer)

- o Note lesions, abnormal discolorations, induration nodules, or ulcerations on or under tongue. Indurated or abnormal lesions may indicate cancer.
- o Inspect for size, shape, color, and papillae.
  - ❖ Loss of papillae: Vitamin B deficiencies, chemotherapeutic agents.
  - ❖ Elongated papillae ("hairy tongue"): Antibiotic therapy, unknown cause (benign condition).
  - ❖ Geographic: Scattered erythematous and denuded patches (benign condition), cause unknown.
  - ❖ Fissured tongue: Benign condition.
  - ❖ Hypoglossal (12th) cranial nerve paralysis: Deviation toward side of paralysis when protruding tongue.
  - ❖ Caviar lesions (varicosities): Small black purplish spots (benign condition).
  - ❖ Leukoplakia: White patches (premalignant).
  - ❖ Carcinoma: Lesions most common at base of tongue or on sides rather than dorsum.

Throat

Examination of the throat is as follows:

- Pharynx:
  - o Use tongue blade to press tongue down and examine the soft palate, pillars (anterior/posterior), uvula, tonsils, and posterior pharynx. Note evidence of tonsillar hypertrophy, infection, or abscess. Erythema, edema, and patches of purulent exudate indicate infection.
  - o Ask patient to say "ahh" and check to see if the soft palate rises to test the 10th cranial nerve.
- Neck:
  - o Inspect neck for masses, scars (thyroid), and symmetry. Note swelling of parotid or submaxillary glands.
  - o Palpate lymph nodes with the head slightly flexed (nodes should be moveable): Pre- and postauricular, occipital, submaxillary, submental, superficial cervical, posterior cervical chain deep cervical chain, and supraclavicular. Note any swelling or tenderness.
  - o Inspect thyroid and cricoid cartilages and trachea, noting deviations from midline and asymmetrical spacing and observing during swallowing (all should elevate).
  - o Palpate the thyroid gland from behind with the patient's neck extended, noting enlargement.
  - o Auscultate enlarged thyroid: Bruit may indicate hyperthyroidism.
  - o Examine carotid artery and jugular veins and evaluate jugular venous pressure. Note pulse intensity and auscultate for bruit (indicating carotid obstruction).

Eyes

Examination of the eyes includes the following:

- Check visual acuity with Snellen eye chart and handheld cards and check visual field with confrontation.
- Note position, alignment, and signs of prominence (bilateral associated with hyperthyroidism and unilateral with tumor).
- Check eyebrows for scaliness and distribution (lateral third loss of hair occurs in normal aging and hypothyroidism).
- Inspect eyelids for ptosis, edema, color changes, lesions.

- Check lacrimal glands and observe for signs of excessive tearing or dryness.
- Note variations and abnormalities in optic disc and retina.
- Note conjunctiva and sclera.
- Yellow sclera may indicate jaundice and pale palpebral conjunctiva anemia.
- Discomfort, itching, redness, and exudate may indicate conjunctivitis. Isolated demarcated red area of conjunctiva indicates subconjunctival hemorrhage.
- Note nonparalytic strabismus: Convergent (esotropia) or divergent (exotropia).
- Note paralytic strabismus:
- Sixth nerve paralysis: Esotropia looking forward with maximum when looking to the side of paralysis, but eyes conjugate when looking to the opposite side.
- Fourth nerve paralysis: The affected eye cannot look down when turned inward.
- Third nerve paralysis. Sixth nerve pulls eye outward, so up, down, and inward movement is impaired. May be associated with dilated pupil and ptosis.
- Ciliary injection (deep vessel dilation causing radiating vessels or flush around limbus) may indicate corneal injury, acute iritis, or acute glaucoma.
- Use oblique lighting to inspect corneas, irises, and lenses. Note signs of glaucoma.
  - Corneal arcus: Gray/white arc at edge of corner may indicate hyperlipoproteinemia or aging, and is common in African Americans.
  - Corneal scar: Superficial gray/white opacity.
  - Pterygium: Triangular hyperplasia of bulbar conjunctiva that may grow across cornea.
  - Cataracts: Opacity of lens (viewed through pupil). Nuclear cataract forms a central gray opacity. Peripheral cortical cataract has a gray spokelike appearance.
  - Floaters: Benign specks or strands in the vitreous humor.
- Note size, shape, symmetry, and reaction, and accommodation:
  - Benign anisocoria: Slight inequality in size with no other abnormalities.
  - Horner's syndrome (impaired sympathetic nerve impulse): Pupil small, regular, reactive to light and accommodation, associated with ptosis.
  - Ocular nerve paralysis: Nonreactive dilated pupil, sometimes associated with lateral deviation and ptosis.
  - Tonic pupil: large, regular with reduced or absent reaction to light and slow accommodation.
  - Argyll Robertson pupil (usually associated with syphilis): Bilateral small, irregular pupils nonreactive to light but normal accommodation.
  - Dilated, fixed: Brain damage, hypoxia, anticholinergic agents and glutethimide poisoning.
  - Small, fixed: Pontine hemorrhage, glaucoma eye drops, and narcotic drugs.
  - Surgical abnormalities: Iridectomy

Ears

Examination of the ears is as follows:

- Examine the auricles and note any ear pain, discharge, or inflammation (movement elicits auricle pain in acute otitis externa, and pain posterior to the ear indicates otitis media).
- Examine the ear canal and eardrum with otoscope noting discharge, cerumen, and foreign bodies. Swelling of the canal is often present with acute otitis externa and thickening occurs with chronic otitis. The eardrum may be red and bulging with otitis media.

- Weber's test may be done to evaluate lateralization and Rinne's test for bone and air conduction.
  - Weber's test: A vibrating tuning fork is touched to the top of the head or the forehead, and the child is asked if the sound is equal in both ears. A hearing deficit in one ear suggests sensorineural hearing loss.
  - Rinne's test: A vibrating tuning fork is held on the mastoid bone, and the time is measured until the sound ceases. Then the vibrating tuning fork is held at the external ear. Sound is normally heard twice as long through air as through bone. If there is conductive hearing loss, the sound is heard longer through the bone. If there is sensorineural hearing loss, the sound is heard longer through the air.

Abdomen

Inspection and auscultation: The abdomen should be examined with the patient in supine position and arms across the chest or at the sides after urinating:

- View tangentially to note contour (flat, round, protuberant, scaphoid) and peristalsis. Evaluate protuberance: Fat (sunken umbilicus common), gaseous distention (tympanic percussion), tumor (dull to percussion), pregnancy (confirm with fetoscope), ascites (bulging flanks dull to percussion with location shifting if patient is positioned laterally).
- Note scars, striae, or dilated vessels and symmetry, position of umbilicus and contour as well as rash, irritation, or hernias.
- Auscultate abdominal sounds:
  - Bruits: Hepatic (carcinoma, alcoholic hepatitis) and arterial (occlusion)
  - Venous hum: Epigastric and umbilical (increased collateral circulation with cirrhosis).
  - Friction rub: Hepatic and splenic (peritoneal inflammation from tumor, gonococcal hepatitis, splenic infarct, post–liver biopsy).
  - Use percussion to measure liver, spleen, and identify abdominal contents.

Palpation: The abdomen should be examined with the patient in supine position and arms across the chest or at the sides after urinating:

- Palpate and note tenderness, rigidity, spasms, tumors, acute peritoneal tenderness:
  - Cholecystitis: RUQ pain (check with Murphy's sign).
  - Pancreatitis: Epigastric tenderness and rebound tenderness with soft abdominal wall.
  - Appendicitis: RLQ pain.
  - Diverticulitis: LLQ (sigmoid lesions).

Liver, spleen, kidneys, and aorta:

- Liver - Palpate by supporting the back with the left hand at ribs 11 to 12 while gently palpating upward from the right abdomen with the right hand. Use percussion to determine shape and palpation to evaluate margins. The normal liver is usually palpable about 4 cm below midclavicular costal margin:
  - Cirrhosis: Enlarged with firm nontender margin.
  - Hepatitis/inflammation/right-sided heart failure: Enlarged with smooth tender margin.
  - Malignancy: Enlarged firm, hard with irregular margin, with or without nodules or tenderness.

- Spleen: Usually not palpable unless it is enlarged. Support the posterior lower left rib cage with the left hand and palpate with the right, palpating for the lower margin of the spleen as the patient takes a deep breath, repeating procedure with the patient in the side-lying position.
- Kidneys: Palpate by pressing upward with the left hand just below the 12th rib posteriorly and downward with the right hand in the right upper quadrant. Note pain (infection) enlargement (cysts, hydronephrosis) or masses (tumor).
- Aorta: Palpate in upper abdomen, slightly left of the midline, and note pulsations and enlargement (≥2 cm).

Assessment of heart sounds

S1 and S2: Auscultation of heart sounds can help to diagnose different cardiac disorders. Areas to auscultate include the aortic area, pulmonary area, Erb's point, tricuspid area, and the apical area. The normal heart sounds represent closing of the valves. The first heart sound (S1) "lub" is closure of the mitral and tricuspid valves (heard at apex/left ventricular area of the heart). The second heart sound (S2) "dub" is closure of the aortic and pulmonic valves (heard at the base of the heart). There may be a slight splitting of the S2. The time between S1 and S1 is systole, and the time between S2 and the next S1 is diastole. Systole and diastole should be silent, although ventricular disease can cause gallops, snaps, or clicks, and stenosis of the valves or failure of the valves to close can cause murmurs. Pericarditis may cause a friction rub.

Additional heart sounds:

- Gallop rhythms:
  - S3 occurs after S2 in children and young adults but may indicate heart failure or left ventricular failure in older adults (heard with patient lying on the left side).
  - S4 occurs before S1 and occurs with ventricular hypertrophy, such as from coronary artery disease, hypertension, or aortic valve stenosis.
- Opening snap - Unusual high-pitched sound occurring after S2 with stenosis of mitral valve from rheumatic heart disease.
- Ejection click - Brief high-pitched sound occurring immediately after S1 with stenosis of the aortic valve.
- Friction rub - Harsh, grating sound heard in systole and diastole with pericarditis.
- Murmur - Sound caused by turbulent blood flow from stenotic or malfunctioning valves, congenital defects, or increased blood flow. Murmurs are characterized by location, timing in the cardiac cycle, intensity (rated from Grade I to Grade VI), pitch (low to high pitched), quality (rumbling, whistling, blowing), and radiation (to the carotids, axilla, neck, shoulder, or back).

Jugular venous pressure

Jugular venous pressure (neck vein) is used to assess the cardiac output and pressure in the right heart as the pulsations relate to changes in pressure in the right atrium. This procedure is usually not accurate if the pulse rate is >100. This is a noninvasive estimation of central venous pressure and waveform. Measurement should be done with the internal jugular if possible; if that is not possible, the external jugular may be used.

- Elevate the patient's head to 45° (and to 90° if necessary) with the patient's head turned to the opposite side of the examination.
- Position the light at an angle to illuminate veins and shadows.

- Measure the height of the jugular vein pulsation above the sternal joint by using a ruler.
  - Normal height is ≤4 cm above the sternal angle
  - Increased pressure (>4cm) indicates increased pressure in the right atrium and right heart failure. It may also indicate pericarditis or tricuspid stenosis. Laughing or coughing may trigger the Valsalva response and also cause an increase.

Breast

Breasts should be observed with the patient disrobed to the waist, arms at sides, arms overhead, and hands against hips (arms akimbo), and leaning forward. Note size and symmetry, contour, color of skin, edema, and venous pattern. Note site, size, and character of nodules. Signs of cancer can include:

- Retraction of fibrotic tissue and flattening of nipple.
- Dimpling of skin, abnormal contours, prominent veins.
- Thickening or edema of skin with enlarged pores, and erythema (peau d'orange).

Examine nipples and areolas for size, shape, direction, abnormalities, rashes, ulcerations, and discharge. Identify supernumerary breasts. Examine axillary lymph nodes for hyperplasia/tenderness. Note abnormalities that may indicate cancer:

- Inversion, flattening, or retraction.
- Deviation in axis of pointing, toward lesion.
- Edematous nipple and areola may indicate lymphatic blockade.
- Discharge (most are nonmalignant).
- Paget's disease of the nipple: Red erosion/ulceration about the nipple.

Male breast: Enlarged tissue under the areola indicates gynecomastia. Breast cancer may present as hard, irregular areolar nodule, often distorting the nipple and areola.

Male reproductive

The male reproductive examination is usually conducted with the patient supine or standing:

- Note: If the patient experiences an erection during the exam, advise him this is a normal response and continue with the examination.
- Note the size and shape of the penis and the presence of foreskin (if present, retract and note phimosis or paraphimosis). Note sexual maturity. Palpate shaft and note abnormalities: hypospadias, chancre, genital herpes, venereal warts, carcinoma, Peyronie's disease.
- Examine the glans for balanitis/balanoposthitis. Note urethral discharge. Examine surrounding tissue for excoriations, nits, or rash.
- Inspect and palpate scrotum and testes, nothing abnormalities: Hydrocele, hernia, nodules, masses, cyst, varicocele, epididymitis, sebaceous cysts, orchitis, torsion, small size (<3.5 cm long), cryptorchidism, and scrotum edema.
- Inspect and palpate for hernias (standing): Direct inguinal (above inguinal ligament and often in the scrotum), indirect inguinal (above inguinal ligament but rarely in the scrotum), and femoral (below inguinal ligament and never in scrotum).

Female reproductive

The female reproductive examination is conducted with the patient draped in the lithotomy position.

- Ask patient to urinate before exam.
- Assess sexual maturity and inspect external genitalia, noting excoriations, nits, rash. Note inflammation, discharge, swelling, nodules, ulcerations, or other lesions.
- Note vulvar lesions: sebaceous cyst, venereal warts, syphilitic lesions (condylomata, chancre), genital herpes, or carcinoma (raised ulcerated red lesions).
- Manually palpate the cervix and inspect for abnormalities: cystocele, rectocele, inflamed Bartholin's gland, prolapse of urethral mucosa, and urethral caruncle.
- Insert speculum and inspect cervix: Nulliparous/parous, lacerations, ectropion, retention cysts, cervical polyps, and carcinoma. Complete Pap smear.

The female reproductive examination is conducted with the patient draped in the lithotomy position.

- Inspect vagina and note abnormalities: Trichomonas (malodorous white-to-green discharge, pruritis, red, mucosa), monilia (white curdlike discharge, itching, red swollen mucosa), gonorrhea (urethritis with greenish-yellow discharge), vaginitis (thin gray malodorous discharge), and atrophic (age-related) vaginitis (discharge varies, but mucosa is dry and atrophied).
- Do bimanual examination and note abnormalities: myomas, prolapse, retroversion, and retroflexion.
- Inspect ovaries and note adnexal masses.
- Insert index finger in vagina and middle finger in rectum and repeat bimanual examination.

AOM

Acute otitis media (AOM) is defined as an infection of the middle ear. The cause is congestion of the Eustachian tube. This congestion prevents the flow of middle ear secretions, thereby promoting the growth of pathogenic organisms. Signs and symptoms may include previous upper respiratory infection, acute ear pain, fever, and decreased hearing. Severe cases may include vertigo, nausea, and vomiting. Diagnostic tests are usually not needed; the diagnosis is based on history and physical examination. Examination may reveal a tympanic membrane (TM) that is bulging, red, and immobile. An air/fluid level may be present, along with preauricular nodes. Management includes antibiotics, decongestants, topical analgesic ear drops, and pain medication. The patient should be instructed to use the Valsalva maneuver several times a day (which may be initially painful) and to return for a follow-up visit in ten days. The patient should be referred to an ENT specialist if several trials of antibiotics yield no improvement.

Conjunctivitis

Conjunctivitis is an inflammation of the conjunctiva due to several medical causes.

- Viral: adenovirus, herpes simplex, and herpes zoster
- Bacterial: many bacteria can be the causative organism
- Allergy: pollen, pet dander, and dust mites. The conjunctivitis is caused by the release of histamine when mast cells degranulate.

- 26 -

Signs and symptoms of viral and allergic conjunctivitis include a gritty feeling in and redness of the eyes, along with a clear discharge. Bacterial conjunctivitis may include pain, photophobia, and mucopurulent discharge. Diagnostic tests that should be considered are fluorescein staining of the eye (dendritic lesions are the hallmark of herpes infection) and culture and sensitivity testing of any mucopurulent discharge. Management is determined by the cause. If herpetic lesions are found, an immediate referral to an ophthalmologist is needed. If allergic etiology is diagnosed, topical antihistamines, topical mast cell stabilizers, or a combination of both may be considered. The patient should be referred to an ophthalmologist if there is no improvement after 48 hours.

Rectal exam

The rectal exam is usually done after the examination of female genitalia with the woman in the lithotomy position to accommodate bimanual palpation. However, a male rectal exam or rectal examination alone for a female is with the patient lying on the left side with knees flexed. Inspect the sacrococcygeal and perianal area for lesions, inflammation, or excoriation. Insert a lubricated gloved finger while the patient bears down to relax the sphincters. Note sphincter tone, tenderness, and induration. Insert the finger further, and palpate right, posterior, and left and then anterior surface. Abnormalities include:

- Pilonidal cyst: Small sinus tract in sacrococcygeal area.
- Anorectal fistula: Open tract from anus/rectum to skin.
- Anal fissure: Painful ulceration in anal canal, often with sentinel skin tag posterior to fissure and spastic sphincter.
- Prolapse: Mucosa only or length of bowel.
- Internal hemorrhoids: Usually not palpable, but rectal exam may elicit bright red bleeding.
- External hemorrhoids. Tender swollen, bluish, masses at anus.
- Rectal polyps: Pedunculated or sessile in varying sizes—may be difficult to palpate.
- Rectal carcinoma: Polypoid or firm and nodular mass.

<u>Extremities</u>

Arterial vs. venous insufficiency:

Characteristic	Arterial	Venous
Type of pain	Ranges from intermittent claudication to severe constant.	Aching and cramping.
Pulses	Weak or absent.	Present.
Skin of extremity	Rubor on dependency but pallor of foot on elevation. Skin pale, shiny, and cool with loss of hair on toes and foot. Nails thick and ridged.	Brownish discoloration (hemosiderin) around ankles and anterior tibial area.
Ulcers	Pain, deep, circular, often necrotic ulcers on toe tips, toe webs, heels, or other pressure areas.	Varying degrees of pain in superficial, irregular ulcers on medial or lateral malleolus and sometimes the anterior tibial area.
Extremity edema	Minimal.	Moderate to severe.

Venous refill, capillary refill, skin temperature: Assessment of perfusion can indicate venous or arterial abnormalities:

- Venous refill time: Begin with the patient lying supine for a few moments and then have the patient sit with the feet dependent. Observe the veins on the dorsum of the foot and count the seconds before normal filling. Venous occlusion is indicated with times >20 seconds.
- Capillary refill: Grasp the toenail bed between the thumb and index finger, and apply pressure for several seconds to cause blanching. Release the nail and count the seconds until the nail regains normal color. Arterial occlusion is indicated with times >2 to 3 seconds. Check both feet and more than one nail bed.
- Skin temperature: Using the palm of the hand and fingers, gently palpate the skin, moving distally to proximally and compare both legs. Arterial disease is indicated by decreased temperature (coolness) or a marked change from proximal to distal. Venous disease is indicated by increased temperature about the ankle.

ABI: The ankle–brachial index (ABI) examination is done to evaluate peripheral arterial disease of the lower extremities.

- Apply blood pressure cuff to one arm, palpate brachial pulse, and place conductivity gel over the artery.
- Place the tip of a Doppler device at a 45° angle into the gel at the brachial artery, and listen for the pulse sound.
- Inflate the cuff until the pulse sound ceases, and then inflate 20 mm Hg above that point.
- Release air, and listen for the return of the pulse sound. This reading is the brachial systolic pressure.
- Repeat the procedure on the other arm, and use the higher reading for calculations.
- Repeat the same procedure on each ankle with the cuff applied above the malleoli and the gel over the posterior tibial pulse to obtain the ankle systolic pressure.
- Divide the ankle systolic pressure by the brachial systolic pressure to obtain the ABI.
- Sometimes, readings are taken both before and after five minutes of walking on a treadmill.

Once the ankle–brachial index (ABI) examination is completed, the ankle systolic pressure must be divided by the brachial systolic pressure. Ideally, the blood pressure at the ankle should be equal to that of the arm or slightly higher. With peripheral arterial disease, the ankle pressure falls, affecting the ABI. Additionally, some conditions that cause calcification of arteries, such as diabetes, can cause a false elevation. Calculation is simple; if the ankle systolic pressure is 90 and the brachial systolic pressure is 120:

- $90 \div 120 = 0.75$

ABI scoring is described below:

> > 1.3 = Abnormally high, may indicate calcification of vessel wall.
> 1 to 1.1 = Normal reading, asymptomatic.
> < 0.95 = Indicates narrowing of one or more leg blood vessels.
> < 0.8 = Moderate, often associated with intermittent claudication during exercise.
> ≤ 0.6 to 0.8 = Borderline perfusion.
> 0.5 to 0.75 = Severe disease, ischemia.
> < 0.5 = Pain, even at rest, limb − threatening condition.
> 0.25 = Critical limb − threatening condition.

Musculoskeletal

A musculoskeletal examination includes assessment of structure and function and ability to perform ADLs.

- Examine individual joints for range of motion and signs of inflammation (edema, rubor, tenderness, erythema), crepitus, and asymmetry.
- Examine surrounding tissue and muscles for nodules, edema, skin abnormalities, and nodules.
- Test muscle strength and stability:
  - Gait: tandem walking (ataxia), walking on heels/toes (distal muscle weakness), hopping in place (weakness, cerebellar dysfunction), show knee bending (proximal weakness of hip and/or knee extensors), rise from sitting (proximal muscle weakness). Note gait disorders (spastic hemiparesis, scissors gait, steppage gait, sensory ataxia, cerebellar ataxia, Parkinsonian gait, and age-associated gait).
  - Abnormal movements: tremors (resting/static, intention, postural, asterixis), tics, choreiform movements, athetoid movements, dystonia, fasciculations, myoclonus, and orofacial dyskinesias.
- Grade reflexes (0 to 4+ scale): Biceps, triceps, supinator, abdominal, knee, ankle, plantar.
- Evaluate abnormal spinal curvature: lumbar flattening, lumbar lordosis, kyphosis, gibbus (angular deformity), list (lateral tilt), and scoliosis.

Peripheral nerve assessment: A musculoskeletal evaluation should include peripheral nerve assessment to determine if injury has impaired nerve function. Nerves function should be assessed for both sensation and movement. Assessment of sensation is done with a sharp or pointed instrument, using care not to prick the skin. The person should feel a slight prick if the sensory function is intact:

- Median - The median nerve branches from the brachial plexus, which arises from C5, C6, C7, C8, and T1. The median nerve travels down the arm and forearm, through the carpal tunnel. Sensation is evaluated by pricking the top or distal surface of the index finger. Movement is evaluated by having the person touch the ends of the thumb and little finger together and having the person flex the wrist.
- Peroneal - The peroneal nerve branches from the sciatic nerve, which arises from the L4, L4 and S1, S2, and S3 dorsal nerves and travels down the leg. The peroneal nerve enervates the lower leg, foot, and toes. Evaluate sensation by pricking the webbed area between the great and second toe. Evaluate movement by having the person dorsiflex and extend the foot.
- Radial - The radial nerve branches from the brachial plexus and enervates the dorsal surface of the arm and hand, including the thumb and fingers 2, 3, and 4. Evaluate sensation by pricking in skin in the webbed area between the thumb and the index finger. Evaluate movement by having the person extend the thumb, the wrist, and fingers at the metacarpal joint.
- Tibial - The tibial nerve branches from the sciatic nerve. The tibial nerve travels down the back of the leg, through the popliteal fossa at the back of the knee and terminates at the plantar side of the foot. Evaluate sensation by pricking the medial and lateral aspects of the plantar surface of the foot. Evaluate movement by having the person plantar flex the toes and then the ankle.

- Ulnar - The ulnar nerve branches from the sciatic nerve and travels down the arm from the shoulder, traveling along the anterior forearm beside the ulna, to the palm of the hand. Evaluate sensation by pricking the distal fat pad at the end of the small finger. Evaluate movement by having the person extend and spread all fingers.

Manual muscle grading: Manual muscle grading assesses muscle strength and endurance and requires experience to determine the amount of resistance to apply and to assess normal muscle force in different positions. Observation of the muscles for size and shape should precede testing, and the examiner should test muscles on both sides to assess the difference. There are a number of different scales, but the most commonly used is Janda's 0 to 5 scale:

- 0: The muscle shows no contractility.
- 1: The muscle contracts slightly, but there is no effective movement.
- 2: The muscle contracts slightly and range of motion is complete if the effects of gravity are eliminated.
- 3: The muscle can go through the complete range of motion against gravity without resistance.
- 4: The muscle has good strength and complete range of motion against moderate resistance.
- 5: The muscle has good strength and complete range of motion against strong resistance.

Cranial nerve assessment

Cranial nerve assessment should be performed as follows:

- Olfactory (smell) - Ask the person to smell and identify a substance, such as coffee or soap, with one nostril held closed and then the other.
- Optic (vision) - Test visual acuity and the ability to recognize color. Test each eye separately. Red desaturation is tested by having the person look at a red object with first one eye and then the next to determine if the color looks the same with both eyes or is dull with one eye.
- Oculomotor (eye muscles and pupil response) - Using a penlight, the examiner checks eyes are checked for size, shape, reaction to light and accommodation. Eyes are checked for rotation and conjugate movements. The lids should be examined for ptosis.
- Trochlear (eye muscles—upward movement) - Check eye movement by having the person follow a moving finger with the eyes on the vertical plane.
- Trigeminal (chewing muscles, sensory) - The person closes his or her eyes for the sensory examination and is instructed to indicate when part of the face is stroked (light stroke with cotton). The forehead, cheek, and jaw are stroked. The same areas are then examined for sharpness or dullness. The eye should be observed for blinking and tearing, but touching the cornea with cotton or other items should be avoided, as it can cause abrasion. The jaw muscles are assessed by having the person hold the mouth open as well as palpating the muscles on each side to determine if they are equal in size and strength.
- Abducens nerve (eye muscles—lateral movement) - Ask the person to follow your finger from the 1 o'clock position clockwise to the 11 o'clock position. At the horizontal and vertical axis, the eyes should be checked for deviation or nystagmus, which may occur normally only in the extreme lateral position.

- Facial nerve (facial expression, tears, taste, and saliva) - Usually, only the motor portion is evaluated for nerve VII, and taste is examined with testing of cranial nerve IX, but one can test the ability to discriminate between salt and sugar. Motor functions are assessed by asking the person to frown, smile, puff out the cheeks, and wrinkle the forehead. The muscles are observed for symmetry. The person is asked to hold the eyes tightly closed while the examiner attempts to open the lids with the thumb on the lower lid and the index finger on the upper lid, using care not to apply pressure to the eye.
- Vestibulocochlear (balance and hearing) - Check balance with tandem gait and Romberg's test. Check hearing (with the person's eyes closed) by rubbing fingers together or holding a ticking watch next to one ear and then the other. Use Weber's test to evaluate lateralization and Rinne's test for bone and air conduction.
- Glossopharyngeal (taste, mouth sensation) - This test is not usually performed unless the person complains of lack of taste or abnormalities of taste. The mouth must be moist for accurate assessment, so the person should drink water if possible before the test and the testing substance should be in solution. Test for recognition of sweet, sour, bitter, and salt.
- Vagus (swallowing, gag reflex) - Ask the person to open the mouth and say "aw." The uvula and palate should elevate equally on both sides. Test the gag reflex if the person reports difficulty swallowing or changes in speech by lightly touching the tongue blade to the soft palate. Some people are hyperresponsive, so accurate testing may be difficult.
- Spinal accessory (muscle movement—sternocleidomastoid, trapezius) - Place hands along the side of the client's face, and ask him or her to turn the face first one side and then the other against resistance to determine if the strength is normal and equal. Then, place hands on the person's shoulders and ask him or her to shrug the shoulders, elevating them upward, against resistance to determine if the strength is normal and equal.
- Hypoglossal (tongue) - Ask the person to stick out the tongue to determine if it deviates to one side, indicating a lesion on that side of the brain. To determine if there is equal strength on both sides of the tongue, a tongue blade is held against the side of the tongue and the person is asked to push against it with the tongue. Both sides are checked to determine if strength is normal and equal.

Endocrine

The endocrine system evaluation depends on a general assessment of data derived from the physical examination and noting patterns suggestive of endocrine disorders:

- Diabetes: Polyuria, polydipsia, and sometimes polyphagia, weakness, weight gain (type 2), weight loss (type 1), fatigue, and blurred vision. Glucose testing of blood and urine should be included in exam if any indication of diabetes is present.
- Cushing's syndrome: Obesity, hirsutism, edema, ecchymoses, and decreased or absent menses.
- Addison's disease: Weakness, weight loss, bronzing of skin, mucous membranes, nausea, vomiting, and postural hypotension.
- Hypothyroidism: Lethargy, cold intolerance, decreased perspiration, dry skin, hair loss, peripheral edema, periorbital edema, constipation, weakness, bradycardia, and impaired memory.
- Hyperthyroidism: Heat intolerance, anxiety, agitation, moist skin, exophthalmos (with Graves' disease), weight loss associated with increased appetite, diarrhea, palpitations, tremor, and muscle weakness.

<u>Skin</u>

The following characteristics of skin should be examined:

- Color - Pale (albinism, vitiligo, tinea, anemia), red (fever, inflammation, alcohol intake, blush) exposure to cold), yellow (jaundice, increased dietary carotene, anorexia, chronic kidney disease), purplish (polycythemia), blue (cyanosis, cold environment, methemoglobinemia), bronze (hemochromatosis), and brown (sun exposure, melasma of pregnancy, Addison's disease, pituitary tumors).
- Moisture - Dryness, sweating, turgor, mobility, oiliness.
- Temperature - Consistency, generalized or local increased warmth.
- Texture - Rough, smooth, thickened, lichenification, atrophy, scar, keloid, excoriation.
- Hair - Texture, quantity, distribution.
- Lesions - Flat (macule, patch), palpable (papule, plaque, nodule, tumor, wheal), fluid filled (vesicle, bulla, pustule), erosion, ulcer, fissure, crust, scale, comedo (blackhead), nevi, cherry angioma, spider angioma, petechiae, ecchymosis, acrochordons (skin tags), actinic keratosis, lentigo (liver spot), cancerous lesions (basal cell and squamous cell carcinoma, melanoma).
- Nails - Normal (160° angle between fingernail and nail base), clubbed (cyanosis), curved (normal variant), spoon (iron deficiency anemia), Beau's lines (transverse depressions related to acute severe illness), paronychia (inflammation about nail bed), and splinter hemorrhages (linear streaks in nail beds, cause nonspecific).

Blood typing

Blood typing determines the individual's blood type based on antigens on the surface of red blood cells. The ABO blood typing system (AKS Landsteiner) is the most common. RBC surface antigens contain carbohydrate chains, and most contain L-fucose, which forms a structure referred to as the H structure, signifying type O blood. If other sugars are attached to the H structure, then people may inherit the A, B, or AB (both) antigens. People develop antibodies toward the antigens that they lack, so donor blood must match that of the recipient. AB blood type is considered the "universal recipient" because people can receive A, B, or AB blood. Type O is no longer considered a "universal donor," and should not be administered to other blood types. Additionally, there are some extremely rare blood types outside the ABO system, many specific to ethnic groups. These people should keep frozen blood on reserve, because matching their blood in an emergency may be impossible. Blood is also typed for RH compatibility.

Antibody screening

Antibody screening of blood identifies antibodies associated with a variety of diseases. The presence of antibody in the blood indicates that the donor has been exposed to or has a disease. Blood banks routinely check the blood for a number of antibodies for different diseases in order to protect the public health. The FDA sets requirements for blood testing, but blood banks may test for more disorders than required based on recommendations by the FDA or other medical organizations. Blood that tests positive for the following diseases is not used for transfusions:

- Hepatitis B
- Hepatitis C
- HIV
- Human T-lymphocytic virus I and II
- Syphilis

- West Nile virus (not FDA required)
- Chagas disease (not FDA required)

Additional tests are also available and may be done as part of diagnostic studies, including antibody tests for cytomegalovirus and sickle cell trait.

Red blood cell tests

Red blood cell tests determine the following values:

- Total RBCs:
  - Males >18 years: 4.5 to 5.5 million per mm^3.
  - Females >18 years: 4.0 to 5.0 million per mm^3.
- Hemoglobin: Red blood cells (RBCs or erythrocytes) are biconcave disks that contain hemoglobin (95% of mass), which carries oxygen throughout the body. The heme portion of the cell contains iron, which binds to the oxygen. RBCs live about 120 days, after which they are destroyed and their hemoglobin is recycled or excreted.
  - Females >18 years: 12.0 to 16.0 g/dl.
  - Males >18 years: 14.0 to 17.46 g/dl.
- Hematocrit: Indicates the proportion of RBCs in a liter of blood (usually about three times the hemoglobin number). Normal values:
  - Females >18 years: 36% to 48%.
  - Males >18 years: 45% to 52%.
- Mean corpuscular volume (MCV): Indicates the size of RBCs and can differentiate types of anemia. For adults, <80 is microcytic and >100 is macrocytic. Normal values:
  - Females >18 years: 76 to 96 μm^3.
  - Males > 18 years: 84 to 96 μm^3.
- Reticulocyte count: Measures marrow production and should rise with anemia. Normal values: 0.5% to 1.5% of total RBCs.

Glucose and hemoglobin A1C laboratory tests

Glucose is manufactured by the liver from ingested carbohydrates and is stored as glycogen for use by the cells. If intake is inadequate, glucose can be produced from muscle and fat tissue, leading to increased wasting. High levels of glucose are indicative of diabetes mellitus, which predisposes people to skin injuries, slow healing, and infection. Fasting blood glucose levels are used to diagnose and monitor diabetes, but many factors (stress, diet, disease) may impact glucose levels:

- Normal values: 70 to 99 mg/dL.
- Impaired: 100 to 125 mg/dL.
- Diabetes: ≥126 mg/dL.

The hemoglobin A1C test provides the average glucose concentration in the blood. Red blood cells survive about 120 days and are exposed to plasma glucose. These glucose molecules combine with hemoglobin A to form glycated hemoglobin. The percentage of glucose found in the hemoglobin represents average glucose levels over a three-month period, a more reliable indicator of blood glucose levels than the fasting blood glucose.

- Normal value: <6%. (6 = 135 blood glucose).
- Elevation: >7%. (7 = 170 blood glucose).

WBC count and differential

White blood cell (leukocyte) count is used as an indicator of bacterial and viral infection. The white blood cell (WBC) count is reported as the total number of all white blood cells.

- Normal WBC count for adults: 4,800 to 10,000.
- Acute infection: 10,000+, 30,000 indicates a severe infection.
- Viral infection: 4,000 and below.

The differential provides the percentage of each different type of leukocyte. An increase in the WBC count is usually related to an increase in one type and often an increase in immature neutrophils, known as bands, referred to as a "shift to the left," an indication of an infectious process:

Cells	Normal	Changes
Immature neutrophils (bands)	1% - 3%	Increase with infection.
Segmented neutrophils (segs)	50% - 62%	Increase with acute, localized or systemic bacterial infections.
Eosinophils	0% - 3%	Decrease with stress and acute infection.
Basophils	0% - 1%	Decrease during acute stage of infection.
Lymphocytes	25% - 40%	Increase in some viral and bacterial infections.
Monocytes	3% to 7%	Increase during recovery stage of acute infection.

Coagulation profile

The coagulation profile measures clotting mechanisms, identifies clotting disorders, screens preoperative patients, and diagnoses excessive bruising and bleeding. Values vary depending on the lab:

Prothrombin time (PT)	10 to 14 seconds	Time increases with anticoagulation therapy, vitamin K deficiency, decreased prothrombin, disseminated intravascular coagulation (DIC), liver disease, and malignant neoplasm. Some drugs may shorten time.
Partial thromboplastin time (PTT)	30 to 45 seconds	Increases with hemophilia A & B, von Willebrand's disease, vitamin deficiency, lupus, DIC, and liver disease.
Activated partial thromboplastin time (aPTT)	21 to 35 seconds	Similar to PTT, but decreases in extensive cancer, early DIC, and after acute hemorrhage. Used to monitor heparin dosage.
Thrombin clotting time (TCT) or Thrombin time (TT)	7 to 12 seconds (<21)	Used most often to determine dosage of heparin. Prolonged with multiple myeloma, abnormal fibrinogen, uremia, and liver disease.

Bleeding time	2 to 9.5 minutes	(Using the Ivy method on the forearm.) Increases with DIC, leukemia, renal failure, aplastic anemia, von Willebrand's disease, some drugs, and alcohol.
Platelet count	150,000 to 400,000	Increased bleeding <50,000 and increased clotting >750,000.

Endocrine hormone function studies

The following are types of hormone function studies:

- Pituitary - Serum levels of pituitary hormones and hormones of target organs, dependent on stimulation by pituitary hormones, are measured to determine abnormalities.
- Thyroid:
    - Thyroid stimulating hormone (TSH) (0.4 to 6.15 μ/U/mL). Increase in TSH indicates hypothyroidism and decrease indicates hyperthyroidism
    - Free thyroxine (FT_4) (0.9 to 1.7 ng/dL). FT_4 is used to confirm TSH abnormalities.
    - Serum T_3 (17 to 20 ng/dL) and T_4 (4.5 to 11.5 μg/dL). These usually increase together, but elevated T_3 more accurately diagnoses hyperthyroidism.
    - T_3 resin uptake (25 to 35%). Increases with hyperthyroidism and decreases with hypothyroidism.
- Parathyroid - Parathormone level (20 to 70 mEq/L) and serum calcium levels (1.15 to 1.34 mg/dL). Both increase with hyperparathyroidism. Calcium level decreases with hypoparathyroidism and phosphate levels (2.4 to 4.1 mEq/L to 6 mEq/L) increase.
- Adrenal:
    - Catecholamine (urine and serum) levels: Epinephrine (100 pg/mL) and norepinephrine (<100 to 550 pg/mL) elevate with pheochromocytoma.
    - Electrolyte and glucose levels.
    - ACTH and serum cortisol levels and ACTH stimulation test to evaluate for Addison's.
    - Dexamethasone suppression test for Cushing's disease.

Reproductive hormone tests

Human chorionic gonadotropin (HCG)

HCG is secreted by the placenta 8 to 10 days after conception with implantation of the fertilized ovum. HCG stimulates the corpus luteum to secrete progesterone. Levels are decreased in ectopic pregnancy and threatened, incomplete, or spontaneous abortion. Normal levels (in mIU/mL):

Nonpregnant = 5
< 7 days = 5 to 50
2 wks = 50 to 500
3 wks = 100 to 10,000
4 wks = 1,000 to 30,000
5 wks = 35,000 to 115,000
6 to 8 wks = 12,000 to 270,000
12 wks = 15,000 to 220,000

Estradiol

There are three types of estrogen in the blood. Estrone is the precursor to estradiol (the most active form). Estriol is secreted in large amounts from the placenta during pregnancy. Normal levels of estradiol (in pg/mL):

- Early follicular phase: 200 to 150
- Late follicular phase: 40 to 350
- Midcycle peak: 150 to 750
- Luteal phase: 30 to 450
- Postmenopause: <20

Progesterone

Progesterone prepares the uterus for pregnancy and the breasts for lactation. Levels may confirm ovulation (in ng/mL):

- Adult: <0.5
- Follicular phase: 0.2 to 1.4
- Luteal phase: 3.3 to 25.6
- First trimester: 11.2 to 90
- Second trimester: 25.5 to 89.4
- Third trimester: 48.4 to 422.5
- Postmenopause: 0.0 to 0.7

Gonadotropin-releasing hormone (GnRH) stimulating test

GnRH stimulates release of FSH and LH from the anterior pituitary. Production varies with the menstrual cycle, increasing prior to ovulation. The GnRH stimulating test identifies excess or deficiency. A normal response to a bolus of GnRH is increased LH (4 to 10 increments).

Follicle stimulating hormone (FSH)

FSH is produced and stored in the anterior pituitary. FSH promotes maturation of the germinal follicle by increasing estrogen secretion and allowing the ovum to mature. FSH levels define phases of the menstrual cycle for fertility testing. Normal results:

- Follicular phase: 1.4 to 9.9 mIU/mL.
- Ovulatory peak: 6.2 to 17.2 mIU/mL.
- Luteal phase: 1.1 to 9.2 mIU/mL.
- Postmenopause: 19 to 100 mIU/mL

Luteinizing hormone (LH)

LH is produced and stored in the anterior pituitary. LH levels increase during the ovulatory phase of the menstrual cycle in response to high estrogen levels, causing the ovum to be expelled from the ovary, development of the corpus luteum, and production of progesterone. Normal results:

- Follicular phase: 1.7 to 15 mIU/mL.
- Ovulatory phase: 21.9 to 56.6 mIU/mL.
- Luteal phase: 0.6 to 16.3 mIU/mL.
- Postmenopause: 14.2 to 52.3 mIU/mL.

Liver function studies

There are many factors to be examined in liver function studies:

- Bilirubin - Determines the ability of the liver to conjugate and excrete bilirubin: direct 0.0 to 0.3 mg/dL, total 0.0 to 0.9 mg/dL, and urine 0.
- Total protein - Determines if the liver is producing protein in normal amounts: 7.0 to 7.5 g/dL:
    o Albumin: 4.0 to 5.5 g/dL.
    o Globulin: 1.7 = 3.3 g/dL.
    o Serum protein electrophoresis is done to determine the ratio of proteins.
    o Albumin/globulin (A/G) ratio: 1.5:1 to 2.5:1. (Albumin should be greater than globulin.)
- Prothrombin time (PT) - 100% or clot detection in 10 to 13 seconds. PT increased with liver disease. International normalized ratio (INR) (PT result/normal average): <2 for those not receiving anticoagulation and 2.0 to 3.0 those receiving anticoagulation. Critical value: >3 in patients receiving anticoagulation therapy.
- Alkaline phosphatase - 17 to 142 adults. (Normal values vary with method.) Indicates biliary tract obstruction if no bone disease
- AST (SGOT) - 10 to 40 units. (Increases in liver cell damage.)
- ALT (SGPT) - 5 to 35 units. (Increases in liver cell damage.)
- GGT, GGTP - 5 to 55 µ/L females, 5 to 85 µ/L males. (Increases with alcohol abuse.)
- LDH - 100 to 200 units. (Increases with alcohol abuse.)
- Serum ammonia - 150 to 250 mg/dL. (Increases in liver failure.)
- Cholesterol - Increases with bile duct obstruction and decrease with parenchymal disease.

Antibody detection

Rubella

Antibody detection of rubella identifies those who have antibodies, indicating current or past infection or vaccination. Women who are pregnant or anticipate becoming pregnant should be tested to determine the risk of developing rubella. Many women are unsure of their vaccination status. The most common test is the enzyme-linked immunosorbent assay (ELISA). Women should always be vaccinated for rubella before becoming pregnant, as exposure to the virus has devastating effects on the newborn. The mother may not experience any symptoms of the disease or only mild symptoms like mild respiratory problems or rash. If the rubella exposure is during the first four to five months of pregnancy, the consequences for the infant are greater. Infants exposed to this virus *in utero* can develop a set of symptoms known as congenital rubella syndrome. This syndrome includes all or some of the following signs and symptoms:

- Intrauterine growth retardation (IUGR).
- Deafness.
- Cataracts.
- Jaundice.
- Purpura.
- Hepatosplenomegaly.
- Microcephaly.
- Chronic encephalitis.
- Cardiac defects.

<u>Hepatitis</u>

Antibody detection of hepatitis includes tests for hepatitis A (HAV), B (HBV) C (HCV), D (HDV), and E (HEV). HDV occurs only with HBV, so it is not usually part of screening. Antibody testing is indicated if a woman has symptoms of hepatitis, such as anorexia and jaundice, to differentiate the type of hepatitis and plan treatment. Routine HBV screening of all pregnant women and all newborns helps to identify those infected with HBV. Infants are routinely immunized. Hepatitis A is short lived and rarely transmitted to the fetus. Hepatitis C is rarely transmitted to the fetus, and of those infected, about 75% clear the infection by two years. Hepatitis E poses the greatest risk to the mother, with a mortality of about 20% during pregnancy and increased risk of fetal complications and death. Hepatitis E is most common in developing countries but is emerging as an increasing problem in developed countries as well.

Autoantibodies

Autoantibodies are antibodies that develop against organs or specific types of tissue because of genetic predisposition, disease, or other environmental trigger. Some antibodies attack a particular organ, such as the thyroid gland, resulting in Grave's disease. Others target tissue found throughout the body, causing widespread disease, such as rheumatoid arthritis. A positive antinuclear antibody (ANA) test is indicative of autoimmune disorders. The extractable nuclear antigen (ENA) test screens for different antibodies and provides information to help identify specific autoimmune disorders. A number of specific tests are available to narrow diagnosis or differentiate autoimmune from other types of disorders, including:

- Rheumatoid factor: Rheumatoid arthritis and Sjögren syndrome.
- Anticitrullinated protein antibody (ACPA): Rheumatoid arthritis.
- Thyroid stimulating immunoglobulins and antithyroid peroxidase: Autoimmune thyroid disorders.
- Antitissue transglutaminase and antigliadin antibodies: Celiac disease
- Smooth muscle antibody (SMA): Autoimmune and chronic hepatitis.
- Antimitochondrial (AMA): Primary biliary cirrhosis.
- Cardiolipin antibodies: Coagulopathy, APAS.

Renal function studies

The following are renal function studies:

- Specific gravity - 1.015 to 1.025. Determines the kidneys' ability to concentrate urinary solutes.
- Osmolality (urine) - 350 to 900 mOsm/kg/24 hours. Shows early defects if the kidneys' ability to concentrate urine is impaired.
- Osmolality (serum) - 275 to 295 mOsm/kg.
- Uric acid - Male, 4.4 to 7.6; female, 2.3 to 6.6. Levels increase with renal failure.
- Creatinine clearance (24-hour) - Male 85 to 125 mL/min/1.73 m^2, Female 75 to 115 mL/min/1.73 m^2. Evaluates the amount of blood cleared of creatinine in 1 minute. Approximates the glomerular filtration rate.
- Blood urea nitrogen (BUN) - 7 to 8 mg/dL (8 to 20 mg/dL >age 60). Increase indicates impaired renal function, as urea is an end product of protein metabolism.
- BUN/creatinine ratio - 10:1. Increases with hypovolemia. With intrinsic kidney disease, the ratio is normal, but the BUN and creatinine are increased.

- Serum creatinine - 0.6 to 1.2mg/dL. Increases with impaired renal function, urinary tract obstruction, and nephritis. Level should remain stable with normal functioning.
- Urine creatinine - Male, 14 to 26 mg/kg/24 hr; female, 11 to 20 mg/kg/24 hr.

Creatinine, creatinine clearance, and BUN

When food is metabolized, it forms creatine, which forms creatinine. The kidneys filter creatinine, and it is excreted in the urine. The body produces creatinine at a steady rate, but with impairment of kidney function, serum levels of creatinine begin to rise while urine levels fall.

- Serum: 0.6 to 1.2 mg/dL.
- Urine: 11 to 20 mg/kg/24 hr.

Urine is collected for 12 to 24 hours and tested to determine how much creatinine the kidneys are able to clear from the blood. A creatinine clearance formula is:

- (Urinary creatinine/serum creatinine) X urinary volume (mL)/[#of hours X 60] = mL/min.

Patients should avoid strenuous exercise for 48 hours before testing begins and should restrict proteins and meat (especially red meat) ≤8 ounces in the 24 hours before the test begins. When protein is metabolized in the liver, urea is produced and then cleared from the blood by the kidneys. An increase in BUN is one indication of impaired kidney function, but it can also indicate circulatory impairment, a high-protein diet, or dehydration. Normal value: 7 to 8 mg/dL (8 to 20 mg/dL >age 60).

Lipid profile

The NIH, NHLBI Report of the National Cholesterol Education Program Expert Panel on Detection, Evaluation, and Treatment of High Blood Cholesterol in Adults classifies total cholesterol, LDL, and HDL to help to determine the need for treatment. Classification includes:

LDL cholesterol:

< 100 = Optimal
100 to 129 = Near optimal
130 to 159 = Borderline high
160 to 189 = High
≥190 = Very high

Total cholesterol:

< 200 = Optimal
200 to 239 = Borderline high
≥240 = High

HDL cholesterol:

< 40 = Low
≥60 = High (optimal)

Triglycerides:

< 150 = Normal

- 39 -

$$150 \text{ to } 199 = \text{Borderline} - \text{high}$$
$$200 \text{ to } 499 = \text{High}$$
$$\geq 500 = \text{Very high}$$

The optimal LDL goal for those with CHD or an equivalent risk is < 100 mg/dL; zero to one risk factor, <160 mg/dL; and more than two risk factors, <160 mg/dL. Those with coronary heart disease or an equivalent risk factor have a risk of having major coronary events at the rate of >20% per 10 years.

Urinalysis

The following characteristics are examined:

- Color - Pale yellow/amber and darkens when urine is concentrated or other substances (such as blood or bile) are present.
- Appearance - Clear but may be slightly cloudy.
- Odor - Slight. Bacteria may give urine a foul smell, depending upon the organism.
- Some foods, such as asparagus, change the odor.
- Specific gravity - 1.015 to 1.025. May increase if protein levels increase or if there is fever, vomiting, or dehydration.
- pH - Usually ranges from 4.5 to 8 with average of 5 to 6.
- Sediment - Red cell casts from acute infections, broad casts from kidney disorders, and white cell casts from pyelonephritis. Leukocytes > 10 per ml^3 are present with urinary tract infections.
- Glucose, ketones, protein, blood, bilirubin, and nitrate - Negative. Urine glucose may increase with infection (with normal blood glucose). Frank blood may be caused by some parasites and diseases but also by drugs, smoking, excessive exercise, and menstrual fluids. Increased red blood cells may result from lower-urinary-tract infections.
- Urobilinogen - 0.1 to 1.0 unit.

Fecal testing

Fecal testing may be completed to assess for GI bleeding, colon cancer, ova, and parasites. Stool specimens should not be contaminated with urine. Tests include:

- Ova and parasites: Smears from a stool sample are examined microscopically for signs of eggs or parasites.
- Fecal occult blood test (FOBT): Small stool samples are usually applied to a card or other material, sometimes with the addition of a chemical, and sent to a laboratory to test for occult blood. This test requires dietary modifications, a high-residue diet without red meat for two days prior to gathering the sample. Aspirin (high dose) and anti-inflammatory drugs should be restricted for a week before testing and preparations containing vitamin C for two days.
- DNA testing: Stool is examined for abnormal DNA that may indicate a malignancy or polyps.
- Fecal immunochemical test (FIT): FIT tests for occult blood but requires no dietary or medication restrictions and may be more accurate in detecting bleeding from the upper GI tract.

Wet mount

Wet mounts are used to detect any organisms that may cause vaginal, cervical, uterine, or vulvar symptoms, such as yeast, *Trichomonas*, or other causes of irritation. The procedure for a wet mount is as follows:

- The patient should not douche, have vaginal intercourse, or use vaginal creams for 48 hours before the office visit.
- Lubricate speculum with water. Avoid lubricating jelly.
- Obtain specimen from walls of vagina with vaginal spatula or broom.
- First specimen should be prepared with saline solution for detection of clue cells, yeast, red or white blood cells, and trichomonads.
- Second specimen should be prepared with potassium hydroxide (KOH) solution for visualization of yeast hyphae or buds.

Pap smear

Papanicolaou (Pap) smear:

- Used to detect the presence of cancerous and precancerous cells on the cervix
- Done annually after patient has had first sexual intercourse, but no later than when the woman reaches the age of 21
- For women 30 or older, a Pap smear can be performed every two or three years under the following circumstances:
    o If the woman has had three consecutive smears with normal results
    o If the woman has no history of HIV infection, AIDS, immunosuppression, or in utero exposure to DES
- Procedure for performing a Pap smear
    o Patient should not douche, have vaginal intercourse, or use vaginal creams for 48 hours before the office visit. To avoid vaginal bleeding, the Pap test should be performed during the middle of the patient's cycle. Lubricate speculum with water. Sample entire squamocolumnar junction with spatula or broom
    o Obtain endocervical sample with cytobrush

GBS cultures

Group B *Streptococcus* (GBS) is the most common neonatal bacterial infection. Many women are asymptomatic carriers. Pregnant women should have a urine culture early in pregnancy and be treated if the culture shows GBS. GBS screening of all pregnant women around 36 weeks of gestation followed by antibiotic treatment of the mother during labor can prevent neonatal infection. The woman should urinate prior to the procedure. She is then placed in the lithotomy position. A sterile culturette swab is used to swab first the vaginal introitus and then the anal sphincter, inserting the swab through the sphincter and using care not to contaminate the vaginal area after removing the swab. The swab is placed in a nonnutritive medium for transport to the laboratory and labeled, including indications for susceptibility testing (such as erythromycin or clindamycin). A mother needs at least four hours' worth of antibiotic treatment for the infant to benefit.

Tests for ruptured membranes

Fern test (amniotic fluid crystallization test)	Obtain a sample of vaginal fluid with a pipette or sterile swab. Place the specimen on glass slide, smearing it into a thin layer. Air dry for about five minutes. Examine under a low-power (10X) microscope for appearance of fernlike crystals.
Nitrazine/pH test	Obtain a sample of vaginal fluid with a pipette. Place one or two drops of vaginal fluid on test strep that contains Nitrazine dye. Check color, which changes according to pH of the fluid: >6.5 indicates ruptured membrane. The pH of normal vaginal fluid is 4.5 to 5.5 and amniotic fluid 7 to 7.5.
AmniSure (detects PAMG-1 concentration)	Shake solvent and place vertically with the cap off. Using a sterile swab, carefully insert it 5 to 7 cm into vagina, leave it in place for one minute, and then carefully withdraw. Insert swab into solvent and swirl in solution for one minute. Remove swab and place AmniSure test strip in solution for 10 minutes. Interpret results—vertical lines appear on the test strip if positive for amniotic fluid.

Colposcopy

Colposcopy is a procedure that uses a binocular microscope to inspect the vagina and cervix to detect suspicious lesions that may require biopsy, such as polyps, genital warts, and other suspicious lesions. The following procedure is used:

- The patient should not douche, have vaginal intercourse, or use tampons or vaginal creams for 24 hours before the office visit.
- Lubricate the speculum with water only.
- Clean the cervix and vagina with a swab.
- Swab the cervix and vagina with acetic acid (vinegar). This will cause any abnormality to turn a whitish color, which will make suspicious areas visible.
- Take biopsy specimen or specimens.
- If bleeding is a problem, apply silver nitrate or Monsel's solution (ferric sulfate solution). Both of these substances have styptic properties.

Diagnostic laparoscopy

Diagnostic laparoscopy is a minimally invasive procedure increasingly used for abdominal surgery to allow the surgeon to visualize the abdominal or pelvic areas to aid in diagnosis and treatment. Laparoscopy involves one or more small incisions. A 0.5 to 2 cm incision is used for the trochar and laparoscope, but smaller ports (incisions) may be used for instruments to assist with the operative procedure. Laparoscopy causes less dysfunction of the diaphragm and faster recovery because of smaller incisions and less manipulation. Laparoscopy is generally contraindicated with bowel disorders (such as obstruction), cardiorespiratory disease, morbid obesity, increased intracranial pressure, and hypovolemia. During the procedure, insufflation to 12 to 15 mm Hg ($\leq$19 mm Hg) is done with CO_2 to distend the abdomen, and a scope with a video camera is inserted. Diagnostic laparoscopy is done under general anesthesia, so preoperative fasting is required. Postoperative nausea and vomiting are common.

Hysteroscopy

Hysteroscopy is usually performed as an outpatient procedure under local, regional, or general anesthesia. A paracervical block may be used for diagnostic hysteroscopy. The procedure usually takes 30 to 45 minutes to complete. The cervical os is dilated, and the hysteroscopy is inserted into the vagina and through the cervical os. Fluid (such as saline or glycine) may be instilled in order to distend the uterine cavity and provide improved visualization. Fluid inflow and outflow should be carefully measured to check for fluid overload from fluid absorption. CO_2 gas can also be used for insufflation but involves increased risk of gas embolism and prevents cleaning of blood and debris. Contact hysteroscopy involves direct visualization only with no fluid distention. Hysteroscopy may be utilized to assist with diagnosis, to locate intrauterine devices, or to provide treatment, such as endometrial ablation, myomectomy, and polypectomy.

Flexible sigmoidoscopy and colonoscopy

Flexible sigmoidoscopy

A scope is used to check for polyps or signs of cancer in the rectum and sigmoid colon. Colon cleansing must be done prior to the test (laxatives and/or enemas) and sometimes one to three days of a liquid diet. Foods/beverages with red or purple dyes must be avoided. The patient lies on the left side, and the flexible sigmoidoscopy with a camera at the end is inserted, inflating the colon with air, and then slowly removed, allowing for removal of polyps, small cancerous lesions, and biopsies.

Colonoscopy

Colonoscopy is often done with conscious sedation after colon prep (as above). Colonoscopy uses a longer flexible scope to check the rectum and the entire colon. Colonoscopy allows for removal of polyps, small cancerous lesions, and biopsies and provides surveillance of inflammatory bowel disease.

With both procedures, patients may experience slight bleeding, but discomfort should be minimal. Perforation of the bowel can occur and result in severe life-threatening infection. Symptoms include severe pain, distended abdomen, fever, and increased rectal bleeding.

X-rays

X-rays are used for diagnosis and evaluation of treatment and to determine correct placement of medical devices. X-rays pass more readily through soft tissue than dense tissue, so dense tissue, which has less radiation exposure, appears as white against the darker background of soft tissue. Therefore, x-rays are most commonly used for evaluation of bones, such as for fractures or dislocations. They may also be used for soft tissue when a disease or disorder alters the density of tissue, such as with pneumonia in the lungs or gallstones, kidney stones, or tumors, although small tumors may go undetected. Different types of tissue have different color gradations. For example, organs with a high fluid content (stomach, liver) appear gray while muscles (which have more fat) appear slightly darker. Spaces filled with air (such as the lungs) appear very dark. X-rays may be used with contrast medium as well to take images of the cardiovascular or GI systems.

Ultrasonography

Ultrasonography is a procedure that uses high-frequency sound waves to determine the internal structure of the body without the use of invasive procedures. Ultrasonography can be used for the following:

- To determine whether a breast, pelvic, or abdominal mass is present and whether it is cystic or solid
- In conjunction with mammography, to evaluate breast masses
- To determine whether products of conception are present
- To determine the thickness of the endometrium
- To determine whether uterine fibroids are present and, if so, to determine their location and their size
- To detect an ectopic pregnancy
- To evaluate ovarian cysts
- To predict ovulation as part of infertility testing
- To evaluate the growth of the fetus
- To detect fetal abnormalities
- To evaluate structural abnormalities such as placenta previa and abruptio placentae
- To quantitatively evaluate amniotic fluid
- To evaluate the umbilical cord by detecting a two- or three-vessel cord

Bone densitometry

Bone densitometry is recommended for all women ≥65 years and for those with high fracture risks beginning at age 60 to assess osteoporosis. Common methods include:

- X-rays: Do not show early stage osteoporosis.
- CT scan: Provides accurate information but is costly and involves high radiation.
- Dual-energy x-ray absorptiometry (DEXA): Highly accurate with very low radiation (the most widely used method).
- Quantitative ultrasound (QUS): Accurate (but less so than DEXA) with no radiation but usually done on the heel or wrist and cannot assess areas of fractures, such as hips and vertebrae.

Once scans, such as DEXA, are complete, the bone density is quantified with a T score. T score represents the number of standard variations from average bone density of young adults. Osteoporosis is diagnosed with a score of -2.

T score:	Bone Density
0 to 1.0	Normal
-1	10% below normal
-2 (Osteoporosis)	20% below normal

Results may also be presented as a Z score, the number of standard deviations from the average bone density for people of the same age.

Endometrial biopsy

Endometrial biopsy may be done for positive Pap smears to determine the cause of abnormal cells or because of risk factors. The woman is placed in the lithotomy position, a speculum inserted, and tissue sampling done. Different methods include:

- Inserting a pipette into the uterus and suctioning a tissue sample from the lining.
- Dilatation and curettage (under regional or general anesthesia).
- Suction with Vabra aspiration.
- Jet irrigation.

Endometrial biopsy may be done during a hysteroscopy. No special preparation is necessary for the endometrial biopsy except urination unless the woman is receiving an anesthetic, for which preoperative fasting is required. If she is not having anesthesia, the woman may take acetaminophen or ibuprofen one-half to one hour before the procedure to reduce discomfort and cramping.

Cervical biopsy

Cervical biopsy is usually done if abnormalities are found on Pap smear or pelvic exam. A number of different procedures are available, depending on the Pap grade:

- Colposcopy with direct biopsy: 3% to 5% acetic acid is applied to the cervix 5 to 10 minutes prior to examination. The binocular stereomicroscope has a light and green filters to highlight abnormal blood vessels. The acetic acid makes abnormal lesions appear white and more evident. A tissue sample is taken, usually with a punch biopsy.
- Punch biopsy: An instrument removes 4 mm cylindrical tissue samples from the cervix.
- Cone biopsy: A cone-shaped wedge of tissue that includes all of the transformation zone and part of the endocervical canal is removed by various means, including the cold knife, laser, large loop excision of the transformation zone (LLETZ), or a loop electrosurgical excision procedure (LEEP). This procedure is usually done under regional, local, or general anesthesia. Bleeding may occur 5 to 10 days following cone biopsy.
- Curettage: An instrument is used to scrape tissue from the endocervical canal

Vulvar biopsy

Vulvar biopsy is indicated for raised, pigmented, malignant-appearing, thick, or enlarging lesions of the vulva or dermatoses that are unresponsive to treatment. The procedure is done with a local anesthetic, usually in the doctor's office with the patient in the lithotomy position. The tissue is prepped with povidone-iodine or other antiseptic. Different procedures include:

- Colposcopy with application of 3% to 5% acetic acid 5 to 10 minutes prior to the biopsy to help isolate the lesion.
- Toluidine blue dye application: In some cases, toluidine blue dye may be applied to the vulvar area because the dye stains some lesions blue, including vulvar intraepithelial neoplasia and vulvar malignancy.
- Instrumental shaving or cutting of the lesion.
- Punch biopsy removes 4 mm cylindrical tissue samples.
- Excision: Larger lesions may be surgically removed.

After the tissue sample is removed, pressure is applied or the open area cauterized with silver nitrate, although removal of lesions >1 cm may require absorbable suturing.

Breast biopsy

Breast biopsy is carried out when a lesion is found in the breast to determine if the lesion is malignant. A number of different procedures may be used, depending on the size and location of the lesion:

- Fine needle aspiration (FNA): Aspiration of a small amount of tissue through needle and syringe.
- Needle (wire) localization biopsy: Lesion position is verified with mammography and a needle with attached wire placed in the breast with the tip at the lesion to guide excision.
- Stereotactic core biopsy: With the patient lying facedown, the breast is compressed between mammogram paddles and x-rays are taken. A computer plots the correct needle placement for a needle biopsy.
- Open surgical excision: Done under local or general anesthesia. Small lesions (≤2.5 cm) are usually removed, but larger lesions are sampled.
- Vacuum-assisted biopsy: Imaging isolates the lesion and a biopsy probe placed. Breast tissue is suctioned into the device, and a tissue sample is cut. Sampling may be repeated multiple times.

Genetic markers

A genetic marker is an abnormal DNA sequence (gene mutation) on a chromosome that identifies a special characteristic, disposition, or disease. Genetic markers are associated with a number of different diseases, so genetic testing has become increasingly important:

- BRCA1 gene mutation (chromosome 17) and BRCA2 gene mutation (chromosome 11): 50% to 85% chance of developing breast and/or ovarian cancer with early onset.
- CEP17 gene mutation (chromosome 17): Associated with poor outcomes with breast cancer treatment but good response to anthracyclines.
- CHEK2 or TP53 gene mutations: Associated with Li–Fraumeni syndrome and high rates of cancer, including breast, brain, osteosarcoma, and leukemia with early onset.
- HER2 gene mutation: Associated with breast cancers that are estrogen/progesterone positive.
- Huntingtin gene mutation (mHTT) (chromosome 4): Huntington's disease.

Much research is currently underway to determine genetic markers for a wide variety of diseases, such as Alzheimer's, cardiovascular disease, and diabetes because once a genetic marker is identified, targeted therapy, such as the monoclonal antibody Herceptin, which is used for HER2-positive breast cancer.

DNA, genes, and chromosomes

DNA stands for deoxyribonucleic acid. DNA is located in the nucleus of the cell and contains the genetic code for each individual. Specific sequences of bases located in the DNA code form specific proteins that regulate cell functions. Genes comprise sequences of base pairs located on DNA strands. Each gene codes for a specific trait. Genes range in size from a few hundred to several million DNA bases. Every person has two copies of each gene, one inherited from each parent. The genes' code for inherited traits is passed on from parents to offspring. Chromosomes are threadlike structures located in the nucleus of each cell. Human cells normally contain 46 chromosomes (23 pairs). Chromosomes are molecules made up of two strands of DNA wrapped around proteins. Each chromosome has a constriction point (centromere) that divides the chromosome into two arms. The short arm is labeled "p," and the long arm is labeled "q."

Karyotype, sex chromosomes, and autosomal chromosomes

A karyotype is the study of an individual's chromosomes. Human chromosomes are arranged in 23 pairs, totaling 46. Karyotyping determines whether the chromosomes are normal in number and gross structure, because abnormalities may aid in diagnosis. Karyotyping may identify a number of different types of chromosomal mutations: deletion, duplication, inversion, insertion, and translocation. Inversions and translocations usually don't cause disease unless the break point disrupts important genetic material. Translocations may result in reduced fertility. Monosomy indicates that one of a pair is missing. For example, 45X (Turner syndrome) is a monosomy indicating that there are only 45 chromosomes and an X is missing. Trisomy indicates an extra chromosome; for example, trisomy 21 (Down syndrome) is caused by an extra 21st chromosome.

Autosomal chromosomes: Pairs 1 to 22. Pairs should be identical and are numbered sequentially depending upon the number of base pairs.

Sex chromosomes: The 23rd pair of chromosomes that determine a person's sex. A male has an XY pair, while a female has an XX pair.

Genetic testing

Genetic testing identifies abnormal genes associated with a genetic disorder, such as cystic fibrosis. Predictive testing identifies genetic disorders that may manifest at a later date (such as Huntington's disease) or an increased risk of developing a disease (such as breast cancer). Referral for genetic testing may be advised for suspected genetic disorder, familial cancer, retinoblastoma, familial adenomatous polyposis (which can cause colon cancer), cystic fibrosis, Huntington's disease, and amyotrophic lateral sclerosis. Identifying those at risk for developing cancer is especially important so that close monitoring and/or preventive measures can be taken. The BRCA1 breast cancer gene has been mapped to chromosome 17q and the gene for BRCA2 on chromosome 13q. People carrying the abnormal gene have an 80% to 90% chance of developing breast/ovarian cancer. These women should be counseled about their options and the importance of close monitoring and surgical options. Tests are not available for all diseases with a genetic component (diabetes, hypertension, pyloric stenosis, spina bifida, psychiatric disorders, and Alzheimer's disease), but more genes are being identified.

Primary Care

Vitiligo

Vitiligo is a congenital or acquired skin condition in which depigmentation occurs because of a loss of melanocytes in local or widespread areas of the skin, so affected areas appear as white patches. Vitiligo is most common in people with dark skin. The depigmented lesions may vary in size and location but are usually symmetric and permanent. Various treatments are used, including attempts to repigment the skin. Corticosteroids may promote repigmentation if applied at the onset of the disorder. Psoralen photochemotherapy with ultraviolet A (PUVA) is the most effective repigmentation treatment but may result in burning of the skin and hyperpigmentation. Special cosmetics and skin stains are available to mask the area, but large areas are difficult to hide. Depigmentation of pigmented skin may be done if >50% of the skin is depigmented to even out the skin color. Monobenzone is used to treat the skin and results in permanent depigmentation. Skin grafts and micropigmentation (tattoos) may also be used.

Psoriasis

Psoriasis is a chronic noninfectious skin condition caused by rapid turnover of epidermal cells and overproduction of keratin, resulting in red, raised, scaly patches of skin. Psoriasis appears to be triggered by a combination of genetic makeup and environmental stressors. Areas of the skin most commonly affected include the scalp, extensor surfaces of elbows and knees, lower neck, and genitalis. Nails are involved in about 25%. Lesions are usually bilateral and symmetric. Guttate psoriasis (scattered teardrop lesions) is related to recent streptococcal throat infection. Onset of psoriasis is usually between ages 15 and 35. Psoriasis may have periods of remission and exacerbation. About 5% develop psoriatic arthritis. Treatment includes:

- Topical agents: Corticosteroids (usually applied with occlusive dressing), coal tar products, medicated shampoos, and nonsteroidal agents (such as calcipotriene and tazarotene).
- Intralesional agents: Triamcinolone acetonide injections into lesions.
- Systemic agents: Oral corticosteroids, methotrexate, hydroxyurea, oral retinoids, and cyclosporine A.
- Photochemotherapy: Psoralen with ultraviolet A (PUVA) or ultraviolet b (UVB) alone or with coal tar.
- Laser: Excimer laser treatments.

Acne

Acne is acute or chronic inflammation of the sebaceous hair follicles on the face and trunk (chest and upper back), believed to be caused by increased sebum and androgen. The sebum blocks the follicular canals, which become inflamed and infected with anaerobic *Propionibacteria*. About 85% of teenagers ages 12 to 15 suffer from some degree of acne, but in some people, acne persists throughout life. Acne must be differentiated from recent outbreaks of folliculitis caused by *Staphylococcus aureus* and community-acquired methicillin-resistant *Staphylococcus aureus* (MRSA). Acne is categorized and treated by grades:

- Grade I: Comedonal acne, treated with Retin-A daily and salicylic acid.
- Grade II: Papulopustular acne, treated with 2.5% benzoyl peroxide and Retin-A twice daily; topical clindamycin, erythromycin, or tetracycline twice daily.

- Grade III: Cystic acne, treated with Retin-A and benzoyl peroxide twice daily and oral antibiotics, such as tetracycline.
- Grade IV: Severe pustulocystic nodular, treated with Accutane.

Folliculitis and impetigo

Folliculitis is bacterial infection of the hair follicles, often on the face, resulting in pustules, erythema, and crusts that are painful and itchy. Recently, there has been an increase in cases of community-acquired methicillin-resistant *Staphylococcus aureus* (MRSA) folliculitis infections. Folliculitis may occur as a primary or secondary infection and may result from chronic nasal colonization of MRSA.

Treatment includes:

- Antibacterial soaps.
- Topical (Bactroban) and oral antibiotics.

Impetigo is a contagious itchy bacterial infection of the skin, commonly on the face or hands, causing clusters of blisters or sores. In adults, it may be associated with poor hygiene or low economic status. Group A streptococcus usually causes small blisters that crust over. *Staphylococcus aureus* usually causes larger blisters that may be bullous and cause lesions 2 to 8 cm in size that persist for months. Treatment includes:

- Avoid itching
- Gently cleanse area with soap and water.
- Apply topical Bactroban three times daily until healed.
- Oral antibiotics in severe cases.

Molluscum contagiosum

Molluscum contagiosum is a mild viral disease of the skin that occurs worldwide and is most common among children and young adults. Signs and symptoms include yellowish, smooth, spherical or hemispherical lesions ranging in diameter from several millimeters to 1 cm. Each lesion has an umbilication at the apex. These lesions are usually asymptomatic but may occasionally itch and become inflamed. The differential diagnosis includes varicella, warts, lichen planus, and epidermal cysts. Management includes monitoring the lesions (they may resolve without treatment), curettage with cautery, and cryotherapy with liquid nitrogen; however, this treatment may cause scarring.

Herpes zoster

Herpes zoster ("shingles") is caused by the varicella zoster virus retained in the nerve cells after childhood chicken pox. The virus remains dormant until it is reactivated, often in older adults who are immunocompromised. Initial symptoms include pain (often severe burning) and redness. Painful blistering lesions then occur along sensory nerves usually in a line from the spine around to the chest although sometimes the head and face are involved. Facial nerve involvement can cause loss of taste and hearing. Eye involvement can cause blindness. The lesions eventual crust over and heal in 2 to 4 weeks, although some have persistent postherpetic neuralgia for 6 to 12 months. The lesions are contagious to those who contact them and have not been immunized or had chicken pox. The herpes zoster vaccine (single dose) is recommended for those ≥60 years old to prevent shingles. *Treatment* for herpes includes analgesia (acetaminophen), acyclovir, Zostrix (capsaicin cream) to reduce incidence of postherpetic neuralgia, and rest.

Scabies

Scabies is caused by a microscopic mite, *Sarcoptes scabiei hominis,* which tunnels under the outer layer of skin, raising small lines a few millimeters long. Mites prefer warm areas, such as between the fingers and in skin folds, but they can infest any area of the body. As the mites burrow, they cause intense itching and subsequent scratching can result in excoriation and secondary infections. Some develop a generalized red rash. Scabies is spread very easily through person-to-person contact, and staff can easily spread infection among patients. Incubation time is 6 to 8 weeks, and itching usually begins in about 30 days, so people may be unaware they are transmitting scabies. Most infestations involve only about a dozen mites, but a severe form of scabies infection, Norwegian or crusted scabies, can occur in the elderly or those who are immunocompromised and usually causes less itching. However, lesions can contain thousands of mites, making this type highly contagious. *Treatment* includes scabicides or oral medication (Ivermectin), antihistamines, and antibiotics for secondary infection.

Venous dermatitis

Venous dermatitis appears on the ankles and lower legs and can cause severe itching and pain, and without treatment to control the dermatitis, it may deteriorate, causing ulcers to form, so treatment is needed to alleviate the symptoms:

- Topical antihistamines to decrease itching and prevent excoriation from scratching. Low-dose topical steroids should be used only for short periods (two weeks) to reduce inflammation and itching only because of the danger of increasing ulceration.
- Compression therapy, usually with compression stockings, to the affected leg to improve overall venous return.
- Leg elevation when sitting to avoid dependency.
- Topical antibiotics, such as bacitracin, as indicated to reduce danger of infection. Oral antibiotics as indicated for systemic infection.
- Hypoallergenic emollients (without perfume), such as petrolatum jelly, to improve the skin's barrier function is a preventive measure that should be used when the acute inflammation has subsided.

Atopic dermatitis

Atopic dermatitis (eczema) is a chronic inflammatory superficial skin disorder that affects about 10% of children. About 75% of these resolve by adolescence, but some adults develop chronic symptoms. Atopic dermatitis is related to allergies and is associated with xerosis, which is dry skin with impaired barrier function.

Signs and symptoms are as follows:

- Chronic dry, scaly, erythematous, circumscribed papular lesions on the neck, behind the ears, and on flexor surfaces of the extremities.
- Lichenification (extremely dry, cracked skin).
- Increased risk of MRSA infection.

Treatment includes:

- Wet compresses soaked in aluminum acetate for weepy lesions.
- Frequent lubrication of skin three to four times daily with hypoallergenic creams, such as Eucerin, Cetaphil, or white petrolatum.

- Topical corticosteroid ointments (1% to 2.5%) for acute flare-ups.
- Antihistamines to reduce itching at night.
- Avoidance of triggers.
- Antibiotics (oral or topical) for infection.

Contact dermatitis

Contact dermatitis is a localized response to contact with an allergen, resulting in a rash that may blister and itch. Common allergens include poison oak, poison ivy, latex, benzocaine, nickel, and preservatives, but there is a wide range of items, preparations, and products to which people may react.

Treatment includes:

- Identifying the causative agent through evaluating the area of the body affected, careful history, or skin patch testing to determine allergic responses.
- Corticosteroids to control inflammation and itching.
- Soothing oatmeal baths.
- Caladryl lotion to relieve itching.
- Antihistamines to reduce allergic response.
- Gentle cleansing of lesions and observation for signs of secondary infection.
- Antibiotics only for secondary infections as indicated.
- The rash is usually left open to dry.
- Avoidance of allergen to prevent recurrence.

Basal cell carcinoma and squamous cell carcinoma

Basal cell carcinoma (BCC), the most common skin cancer, usually results from sun damage and appears on the head or neck. The initial lesion may have a waxy, translucent appearance with surface vessels evident, although some appear yellow or gray. As BCC grows, the lesion ulcerates and crusts over. Basal cell carcinoma rarely metastasizes. Treatment includes laser therapy, cryotherapy, chemotherapy, and excision (for larger lesions).

Squamous cell carcinoma (SCC), the second most common skin cancer, has a 3% to 4% risk of metastasis that increases in immunocompromised patients. SCC is also related to sun damage and occurs in areas exposed to sun, such as the head, neck, shoulders, and extremities. Lesions often appear wartlike initially but may have varied appearances and may be difficult to differentiate from BCC by appearance alone. Lesions usually ulcerate, crust, and bleed. Treatment is excision and may be followed by radiation, especially if the SCC is large or fast growing.

Melanoma

Melanoma is an aggressive form of skin cancer, resulting in 2% of all cancer-related deaths. Melanomas arise from melanocytes in the skin or other parts of the body and are directly related to sun exposure. Lesions that are >1.5mm thick or with spread to local lymph nodes have a poor prognosis, so early diagnosis is critical. The most common site for melanoma in women is the leg. Women with dark skin also may develop melanomas in the nail beds, palms, and soles of the feet.

Melanoma may develop from nevi (moles), so all nevi should be examined yearly for indications of melanoma:

- Asymmetry.
- Uneven borders (scalloped, notched).
- Color variations in a single mole.
- >6 mm diameter.
- Evolving changes in appearance, size, and color.

Four primary types of melanoma include superficial spreading, lentigo maligna, nodular, and acral lentiginous melanoma. Melanoma can occur at any age. Treatment includes primary excision, evaluation of lymph nodes, adjuvant therapy (chemotherapy and immunotherapy), and radiotherapy.

Allergic rhinitis

Allergic rhinitis is an inflammation of the nasal membranes due to exposure to specific allergens. Such exposure results in the production of IgE antibodies, which in turn causes release of histamine resulting in sneezing, itching, and nasal discharge. Allergic rhinitis can occur seasonally when trees, grasses, and ragweed are present, and perennially with exposure to cockroaches, dust mites, and mold. Signs and symptoms include nasal congestion, clear rhinorrhea, sneezing, itching, sore throat, and cough due to chronic postnasal drip. Physical examination may reveal a pale, boggy nasal mucosa; thin, clear rhinorrhea; red conjunctiva; and dark discoloration beneath both eyes ("allergic shiners"). Diagnostic tests may include a nasal smear to verify the presence of eosinophils and skin testing for the determination of specific allergens.

Pharmacological treatment may include the following:

- Antihistamines: these drugs are more effective if taken before the onset of symptoms. Adverse effects of first-generation antihistamines (Benadryl, Chlor-Trimeton, Dimetapp) may include drowsiness, dry mouth, sedation, and paradoxical CNS stimulation. These adverse effects are minimized or eliminated in the second- and third-generation antihistamines (Zyrtec, Claritin, Allegra)
- Decongestants: these drugs may be combined with antihistamines for more effective control of symptoms.
- Nasal steroids (Rhinocort, Flonase): these drugs have an anti-inflammatory effect and should be used regularly.
- Mast cell stabilizers (Nasalchrom): these drugs prevent the release of antihistamine by preventing the degradation of mast cells.
- Leukotriene receptor antagonists (Singulair): these drugs block the release of leukotrienes.
- Nonpharmacological management includes the removal of items that may become dusty, such as feather pillows, carpets, stuffed animals, and curtains. Daily vacuuming, the use of air conditioning, and the restriction of pet exposure may help.

The patient should be referred to an allergist if symptoms persist.

Pharyngitis

Pharyngitis is an inflammation of the pharyngeal mucosa, usually due to viral or bacterial causes. The signs and symptoms may include throat pain, fever, general malaise, cough, headache, and myalgias. Physical examination findings of viral pharyngitis include a mild redness with little or no exudate. Findings of bacterial pharyngitis include marked redness, positive exudate, and cervical lymphadenopathy. The differential diagnosis of pharyngitis includes peritonsillar abscess, mononucleosis, oral candidiasis, diphtheria, and epiglottitis. Diagnostic tests include a rapid strep throat culture and a bacterial throat culture for detection of bacterial pathogens. Management is based on the diagnosis. If viral etiology is diagnosed, no treatment may be needed except for hydration, bed rest, and topical anesthetic gargles (lidocaine). If bacterial infection is present, antibiotic therapy is indicated. If peritonsillar abscess or epiglottitis is diagnosed, an immediate referral to an ENT specialist is needed.

Sinusitis

Sinusitis is an inflammation or infection of the mucosa of the sinuses. Sinusitis may be characterized as acute or chronic. Acute sinusitis presents with nasal congestion, periorbital pain, headache, fever, and yellowish/green nasal discharge. Facial pain increases when the patient bends at the waist. The sinusitis may also be accompanied by URI symptoms. Chronic sinusitis is a sinusitis that lasts longer than 30 days and is accompanied by nasal congestion, dull headache, postnasal drip, and cough. Physical examination may reveal a mucopurulent nasal discharge, yellowish/green postnasal drip, boggy nasal mucosa, and pain when sinuses are palpated. Radiography of the sinuses may show thickened mucosa, opacity of the sinuses, and air-fluid levels. Management includes antibiotics, decongestants, saline nasal spray, bed rest, and smoking cessation. If nasal vasoconstrictors are prescribed, they should be used for no more than five days to prevent rebound congestion.

Asthma

Asthma is a chronic inflammatory disease of the smaller airways, associated with mucus production and airway constriction. Asthma may be triggered by pollen, molds, dust, dust mites, cockroaches, animal dander, food additives, feather pillows, cigarette smoke, URI, emotional upset, or pregnancy. Signs and symptoms may include wheezing, shortness of breath (SOB), chest tightness, and cough. Symptoms generally become worse at night or on windy days. Physical examination may reveal wheezing, diminished breath sounds, swelling of the nasal mucosa, and atopic skin manifestations such as eczema. Nonpharmacological management includes avoiding known triggers and using air conditioning and air filters. Pharmacological management includes the use of short-acting β_2-agonists such as albuterol if symptoms are mild. If symptoms persist or become more severe, a combination steroid/long acting β_2-agonist, such as fluticasone/salmeterol (Advair), may be added. If symptoms are not well managed in the primary care setting, referral to an asthma specialist is warranted.

Pneumonia

Pneumonia is defined as an acute infection of the lower respiratory tract that is associated with altered breath sounds. Pneumonia may be caused by bacterial, viral, or fungal infection. Risk factors include smoking, previous URI, immunosuppression, and corticosteroid use. Signs and symptoms may include cough, fever, sputum production, chills, dyspnea, and headache. Such symptoms may be masked in the elderly, the very young, and those who are immunosuppressed. Physical examination may reveal tachycardia, tachypnea, dullness with percussion over the affected area of the lung, rales, rhonchi, and diminished breath sounds over the affected area. Diagnostic tests may include chest radiograph; Gram's stain, culture, and tests for sensitivity of sputum; and CBC. Management depends on the diagnosis. If viral etiology is suspected, management of symptoms with cough suppressant/expectorant may be needed. If bacterial etiology is suspected, antibiotics should be prescribed. If there is no improvement within 48 hours, or if symptoms worsen, hospitalization may be considered.

Acute bronchitis

Acute bronchitis is an inflammation of the bronchial tree in which swelling and exudate cause a partial obstruction that prevents the lung from fully inflating. Causes include viruses (most common), bacteria, yeasts and fungi, and noninfectious things, such as smoke or air pollutants. In adults, the most common viral triggers are influenza virus, adenovirus, and respiratory syncytial virus (RSV). Symptoms vary but may include:

- Dyspnea and tachypnea.
- Cyanosis.
- Heavy productive moist or raspy cough.
- Sputum is clear, white, yellow, green, or bloody.
- Localized crackling rales and expiratory high-pitched sibilant wheezes.
- Fever may or may not be present, but prolonged or high fever may indicate a bacterial infection.

Since most cases of acute bronchitis are caused by viruses and are self-limiting in two to three weeks, antibiotics are not helpful, but treatment may include:

- Bronchial dilators (albuterol) to improve air exchange.
- Cough suppressant and/or expectorants to relieve cough.
- Antihistamines for those with allergic triggers.
- Antibiotics for bacterial infections.

Hypertension

Hypertension (HTN) is defined as a systolic blood pressure (BP) of 140 or higher, a diastolic reading of 90 or higher, or both. Cardiovascular risk factors of hypertension include smoking, obesity, lack of exercise, hyperlipidemia, diabetes, aging, and family history. Hypertension is divided into two types – primary (essential) and secondary. Primary HTN has no discernable cause, whereas secondary is due to an underlying pathology. About 90% of HTN cases are primary and the rest are secondary. HTN is usually associated with no signs and symptoms, unless there is a secondary cause. Chronic HTN may be associated with target organ damage (TOD) such as CAD, TIA, or stroke. TOD can include retinopathy, heartbeat irregularities, and decreased peripheral pulses. The differential diagnosis includes thyroid disease, renal disease, drug abuse, OTC "cold medications," and pheochromocytoma. To rule out secondary causes, the following tests should be ordered: UA, CBC, TFTs, glucose level measurement, and EKG.

The pharmacological and nonpharmacological management of hypertension are as follows:

- Nonpharmacological methods include losing weight if obese, increasing cardiovascular and resistance training, decreasing sodium intake, increasing intake of fruits and vegetables, decreasing intake of fats, stopping smoking, and minimizing alcohol intake.
- Pharmacological methods include the use of thiazide diuretics, angiotensin-converting enzyme (ACE) inhibitors, angiotensin receptor blockers (ARBs), calcium channel blockers (CCBs), and beta blockers. Many if not most hypertensive patients will require two or more medications to bring their blood pressure under control.

- The patient should be taught that the problem with high blood pressure will need lifetime management, that no symptoms will be present, that adhering to treatment is important for reducing morbidity and mortality rates; and that compliance with follow-up tests and clinical visits is necessary.
- Referral is indicated for evaluation of secondary causes. The patient should also be referred if a three-drug treatment regimen does not produce the desired response.

Thromboembolic disease

Thromboembolic disease is an obstruction of venous flow associated with clotting and inflammation. It is classified as deep vein thrombosis (DVT) or superficial thrombophlebitis. DVTs usually occur as blood clots that form in the deep plexus of veins in the calf, popliteal, femoral, or iliac veins. If thigh veins are involved, there is a 40% chance that the embolus may migrate to the pulmonary circulation. Superficial thrombosis usually occurs in varicosed veins. Risk factors include recent surgery, immobility, advanced age, cancer, pregnancy, congestive heart failure (CHF), recent myocardial infarction (MI), and obesity. Signs and symptoms of DVT or thrombophlebitis include unilateral leg pain associated with swelling, redness, and warmth. Pulmonary embolus may present with chest pain and shortness of breath (SOB); physical examination may reveal cyanosis, cough, hemoptysis, tachycardia, and fever.

Heart murmur

The differential diagnosis of a heart murmur is based on differentiating an innocent murmur from a pathologic murmur. Tests that may be ordered include electrocardiography to determine the severity and to locate any heart or valvular lesions, chest radiograph to determine any enlargement of the heart, complete blood count (CBC) to rule out anemia, and thyroid function tests (TFTs) to rule out hypothyroidism or hyperthyroidism. Management is based on the findings of physical examination and the results of laboratory tests. An asymptomatic low-grade systolic murmur that is accompanied by negative findings from physical examination and diagnostic testing can be presumed to be innocent and should be followed up. Bacterial endocarditis prophylaxis may be considered, especially if the patient has any cardiac abnormalities or prosthetic heart valves. Two grams of amoxicillin should be given one hour before dental procedures. Any patient with a diastolic murmur or any suspected pathology should be referred to a cardiologist.

Dyslipidemia and metabolic syndrome

Dyslipidemia is defined as increased serum concentrations of cholesterol, low-density lipoproteins (LDLs), and/or triglycerides, and low concentrations of high-density lipoproteins (HDLs). Any combination of these factors can lead to possible coronary heart disease. Dyslipidemia includes any of the following:

- LDL >130 mg/dL
- Triglycerides >200 mg/dL
- HDL <40 mg/dL

Metabolic syndrome includes any three of the following:

- Waist circumference >40 inches in men and >35 inches in women
- Triglycerides >150 mg/dL
- HDL <40 mg/dL in men and <50 mg/dL in women

- Blood pressure >130/85 mm Hg
- Fasting glucose concentration >110 mg/dL

Risk factors include smoking, hypertension, and any family history of heart disease. Dyslipidemia has no signs or symptoms.

The differential diagnosis (DDx) of deep vein thrombosis (DVT) includes muscle strain, cellulitis, contusion, or popliteal (Baker's) cyst. The differential diagnosis of pulmonary embolus (PE) includes MI, pneumothorax, bronchitis, and pneumonia. Management of superficial thrombophlebitis includes warm compresses and pain relief, such as anti-inflammatory medication. The patient should be instructed to avoid sitting for long periods of time and to use support hose to prevent further clot formation. Tests needed for DVT may include duplex ultrasound and contrast venography. Pulmonary embolus evaluation may include perfusion lung scan, arterial blood gases (ABGs) measurement, electrocardiography, chest radiography, and pulmonary angiography. Management of DVT or PE requires immediate referral to the appropriate specialist.

Coronary artery disease

Coronary artery disease (CAD) is defined as atherosclerotic changes to the coronary vasculature, with a resultant decrease in flow because of obstruction. Risk factors include smoking, hypertension, dyslipidemia, diabetes, obesity, and a sedentary lifestyle. Signs and symptoms may include the following:

- May be asymptomatic
- Angina pectoris - Discomfort in the jaw, chest, shoulder, back, or arm, precipitated by stress or excitement, and relieved with nitroglycerine
- Palpitations

The differential diagnosis includes MI, PE, pneumonia, pneumothorax, reflux, peptic ulcer, costochondritis, muscle strain, anxiety, aortic dissection, and shingles prodrome. Tests may include electrocardiography, treadmill testing, myocardial perfusion imaging, and coronary angiography. Nonpharmacological management includes smoking cessation, weight loss, and exercise. Pharmacological management includes treatment of hypertension, diabetes, and dyslipidemia; daily aspirin; nitroglycerine for acute episodes; beta blockers; and long-acting nitrates.

Pulmonary embolism

Clinical manifestations of acute pulmonary embolism (PE) vary according to the size of the embolus and the area of occlusion.

Symptoms include:

- Dyspnea with tachypnea
- Tachycardia
- Anxiety and restlessness
- Chest pain
- Fever
- Rales
- Cough (sometimes with hemoptysis)
- Hemodynamic instability

Diagnostic tests include:

- ABG analysis may show hypoxemia (decreased PaO2), hypocarbia (decreased PaCO2) and respiratory alkalosis (increased pH).
- D-dimer (will show elevation with PE).
- ECG may show sinus tachycardia or other abnormalities.
- Echocardiogram can show emboli in the central arteries and can assess the hemodynamic status of the right side of the heart.
- Chest x-ray is of minimal value.
- Spiral CT may provide definitive diagnosis.
- V/Q scintigraphy can confirm diagnosis.
- Pulmonary angiograms also can confirm diagnosis.

Medical management

Medical management of pulmonary embolism starts with preventive measures for those at risk, including leg exercises, elastic compression stockings, and anticoagulation therapy (Coumadin). Most pulmonary emboli present as medical emergencies, so the immediate task is to stabilize the patient. Medical management includes:

- Oxygen to relieve hypoxemia.
- Intravenous infusions.
- Dobutamine (Dobutrex) or dopamine (Intropin) to relieve hypotension.
- Cardiac monitoring for dysrhythmias.
- Medications as indicated: digitalis glycosides, diuretic, and antiarrhythmics.
- Intubation and mechanical ventilation may be required.
- Analgesia (like morphine sulfate) or sedation to relieve anxiety.
- Anticoagulants to prevent recurrence (although they will not dissolve clots already present), including heparin and warfarin (Coumadin).
- Placement of percutaneous venous filter (Greenfield) in the inferior vena cava to prevent further emboli from entering the lungs may be done if anticoagulation therapy is contraindicated.
- Thrombolytic therapy, recombinant tissue-type plasminogen activator (rt-PA) or streptokinase, for those severely compromised, but these treatments have limited success and pose the danger of bleeding.

Hyperlipidemia

Hyperlipidemia is increased blood levels of lipids, lipoproteins, and triglyceride. Lipoproteins include high-density lipoproteins (HDL), low-density lipoproteins (LDL), and very low density lipoproteins (VLDL). Most triglyceride is found in VLDL particles, so the VLDL fraction can be estimated by dividing the triglyceride level by 5 (if triglyceride level is <400). Elevated triglycerides are associated with atherosclerosis and pancreatitis. Hyperlipidemia may result from genetic disorders, such as familial hypercholesterolemia, and medication, such as protease inhibitors. A common cause of hyperlipidemia is diabetes mellitus (DM). Lipoproteins, like plasma glucose, are dependent on insulin, so poorly controlled type 1 DM may result in increased LDL and triglycerides, but levels may return to normal when disease is controlled. In type 2 DM however, hyperlipidemia is a characteristic of insulin resistance, resulting in elevated triglycerides (300 to 400 mg/dL), HDL <30 mg/dL, and changes in the character of LDL particles (smaller dense particles). A low level of HDL is a risk factor for vascular disease. Treatment includes a low-carbohydrate/low-fat diet, omega-3 fish oil, fibrates, and statins.

Mitral valve prolapse

Mitral valve prolapse (MVP) is a usually asymptomatic abnormality of the mitral valve that occurs in about 3% of reproductive-age women. MVP is usually related to an inherited connective tissue abnormality that results in enlargement of one or both leaflets of the valve and often elongation of the chordae tendineae and papillary muscles. During systole, part of one or both leaflets may prolapse back into the left atrium. This may stretch the leaflets so that some regurgitation may occur. Regurgitation occurs when the mitral valve fails to close completely so that there is backflow into the left atrium from the left ventricle during systole, decreasing cardiac output. MVP is characterized by midsystolic click and late systolic murmur. Some people may experience anxiety, lightheadedness, dizziness, palpitations, syncope, and chest pain. Patients should avoid caffeine, alcohol, and smoking. Treatment includes nitrates for chest pain or calcium channel blockers or beta blockers. In advanced disease, mitral valve replacement may be indicated. Most women with MVP tolerate pregnancy well but are given antibiotic prophylaxis during labor and the early postpartum period to prevent endocarditis.

Digestion, metabolism, elimination, and nutrients (large bowel)

Right-sided (ascending) colon cancer

With ascending colon cancer (the most common type), stool enters the cecum and ascending colon in liquid form, so cancers arising in these areas may grow to a large size before they cause obstruction and obvious symptoms. Lesions frequently grow into the lumen of the intestine and ulcerate, causing chronic bleeding that may not change the character or the appearance of stool. Liquid stool can pass through even a very narrow opening. Twenty-two percent of colorectal tumors arise in the ascending colon. Symptoms include:

- Fatigue, generalized weakness.
- Pallor.
- Dull abdominal pain.
- Anorexia, unexplained weight loss.
- Occult blood or melena (tarry stools).
- Hypochromic microcytic anemia.
- Chronic iron deficiency anemia.
- Palpitations or congestive heart failure related to anemia.
- Palpable abdominal mass may be evident with large tumors.
- Chronic diarrhea may rarely develop with some large right-sided lesions.
- Obstruction may occur in late stages.

Transverse, descending, sigmoid, and rectal cancers

Because some of the fluid in the intestines is absorbed in the ascending colon, stool in the transverse and descending colon is more formed. Lesions arising in the transverse and descending colon tend to be annular constrictive lesions, encircling the intestine and leading to obstruction.

Sigmoid and rectal tumors may cause pressure on adjacent structures, such as the vagina, prostate, and bladder.

Transverse/descending cancers	Sigmoid/rectal cancers
Change in bowel habits may become evident. Abdominal cramping, especially left lower quadrant pain. "Pencil" stools from narrowing of lumen. Constipation. Abdominal distention. Intestinal obstruction. Perforation of bowel/ peritonitis.	Tenesmus (painful, ineffective straining to pass stool). Pain in rectal or perianal area. Feeling of fullness and incomplete evacuation of stool after bowel movement. Alternating constipation and diarrhea. Frank blood in stool, possibly blood clots. "Pencil" thin stools from narrowing of lumen. Abdominal pain and cramping. Urinary symptoms. Vaginal fistula.

GERD

Gastroesophageal reflux disease (GERD) is defined as the movement of gastric contents into the esophagus. If this movement continues, inflammation can occur and can lead to strictures and esophagitis. Risk factors include high-fat foods, chocolate, peppermint (each of which lowers the pressure of the lower esophageal sphincter [LES]), cigarette smoking, alcohol, pregnancy, and obesity. Signs and symptoms may include "heartburn" (defined as a retrosternal burning sensation that radiates upward) and acid regurgitation (defined as the effortless return of gastric contents into the pharynx). Hoarseness, chronic cough, asthma, hiccups, dental disease, and nausea can be symptoms of GERD. The findings of physical examination are usually normal. Management includes losing weight, smoking cessation, elevating the head of the bed, sitting upright for three hours after eating, and reducing the intake of foods known to trigger symptoms. Pharmacological management includes H_2-receptor agonists, such as famotidine and ranitidine, and proton pump inhibitors, such as lansoprazole. The patient should be referred to a gastroenterologist if symptoms persist or if dysphagia or weight loss occurs.

Irritable bowel syndrome

Irritable bowel syndrome (IBS) is a functional disorder characterized by alternating bouts of diarrhea and constipation, associated with abdominal pain. According to the Rome criteria, a diagnosis of IBS is suggested by the following:

- At least 12 weeks of unexplainable abdominal pain within the last 12 months
- Two of the following:
  - o Relief of abdominal pain with bowel movement
  - o Onset associated with diarrhea or constipation
  - o Onset associated with change in form of stool

Including the Rome criteria, signs and symptoms may include bloating, incomplete evacuation, and fecal urgency. The following symptoms are cause for concern: new onset of disease in patients older than 50 years; pain or diarrhea that interferes with sleep; fever; anemia; blood in stool; and weight loss. The physical examination is generally unremarkable except that there may be LLQ tenderness upon palpation.

Nonpharmacological management of IBS includes reassuring the patient that the process is benign; decreasing the intake of caffeine, alcohol, fatty foods, and foods containing sorbitol; and limiting dairy intake if dairy foods increase the severity of symptoms. The patient should also increase fiber intake and exercise. Stress management may also be considered if stress is an issue. Pharmacological management depends on the presentation. If pain predominates, an anticholinergic such as dicyclomine HCl (Bentyl) may be prescribed. Another option would be one of the tricyclic antidepressants, such as amitriptyline or nortriptyline. If the problem of diarrhea is predominant, loperamide (Imodium) may control symptoms. If the predominant problem is constipation, bulk-forming agents, such as Metamucil, may control the problem. The patient should be referred if any of the following are present: onset in patients older than 50 years, or other symptoms that may be suspicious.

Diarrhea

Diarrhea is defined as increased frequency or fluidity of the stool. Acute diarrhea (lasting less than two weeks) can be caused by viruses, protozoa, bacteria, or medications. Chronic or recurrent diarrhea may be caused by protozoa, inflammatory conditions (ulcerative colitis, Crohn's disease), medications, functional problems (irritable bowel syndrome), malabsorption (sprue, lactase deficiency), or systemic disease (diabetes, hyperthyroidism); it may also occur after surgery. Signs and symptoms include abrupt onset, increased frequency of defecation, fluid stools, abdominal cramping, and dehydration if severe. Physical examination may reveal increased bowel sounds and an abdomen tender to palpation. If diarrhea has lasted less than two weeks and there is no blood in the stool, symptomatic treatment is all that is needed. If diarrhea lasts more than two weeks or there is blood in the stool, a stool specimen should be evaluated for leukocytes, occult blood, bacterial pathogens, ova and parasites, and fat content. Blood tests may include TFTs, tests for glucose concentration and HIV, and CBC.

The management of diarrhea is based on the cause. If diarrhea has lasted less than two weeks and no blood is present, antimotility agents, such as Imodium or Lomotil, may be prescribed. These medications may cause sleepiness and anticholinergic side effects such as dry mouth. Other medications that may be considered for diarrhea lasting less than two weeks are antisecretory agents, such as Pepto-Bismol. The patient needs to be told that bismuth preparations may cause a darkened tongue or stool. If a pathogen is identified in the laboratory tests, then the appropriate medication should be prescribed. The patient should be referred to a gastroenterologist if stools contain blood, if the patient has severe abdominal pain, if the symptoms increase in severity, or if an underlying pathology is found.

Constipation

Constipation is defined as a decrease in the frequency of defecation. The etiology of constipation may include diet, adverse effects of medications, structural abnormalities of the GI tract, neurological disorders of the GI tract, and psychological disorders. Signs and symptoms are based on the patient's history. Some patients have a bowel movement two or three times each day, whereas others may have a bowel movement every three or four days. It is the change in the number of bowel movements that defines constipation. Physical examination may reveal a hard stool in the rectum and normal or decreased bowel sounds. Melena, nausea/vomiting, rectal pain, fever, or new onset in a patient older than 50 years are causes for concern and require further workup. Nonpharmacological management includes increasing fluid intake, prune juice, high-fiber diet, and exercise. Pharmacological methods include the use of bulk-forming agents (Metamucil), stool softeners (Colace, Surfak), or laxatives such as bisacodyl (Dulcolax) or milk of magnesia. Refer the patient to a gastroenterologist if any pathology is suspected.

Hemorrhoids

Hemorrhoids are defined as varicosities of the anus or rectum. If a clot forms in the varicosity, it is termed a "thrombosed" hemorrhoid. Hemorrhoids above the anorectal line are categorized as internal; those below the anorectal line are considered external. Hemorrhoids are thin-walled, dilated blood vessels that are engorged with blood. The engorgement increases with increased intra-abdominal pressure, such as during a difficult bowel movement or during childbirth. Risk factors include constipation, pregnancy, a low-fiber diet, and the loss of muscle tone as one ages. Signs and symptoms of internal hemorrhoids include painless, bright red blood on stool; those of external hemorrhoids include itching, pain, and bleeding. Skin tags may be present on the anus; these are the remains of previously thrombosed hemorrhoids.

The findings of physical examination may be normal with internal hemorrhoids (unless thrombosed) and may reveal bluish dilated vessels with external hemorrhoids. A thrombosed external hemorrhoid will appear bluish and shiny and will be exquisitely painful. Tests ordered should include anoscopy and other testing to rule out any suspected pathology. Nonpharmacological management includes increased intake of dietary fiber, exercise, sitz baths, and witch hazel pads for hygiene. Pharmacological management includes topical anesthetics or suppositories, bulk-forming agents (Metamucil), and stool softeners. Patient education includes discussions of increased intake of dietary fiber, exercise, and proper use of laxatives. The patient should be referred to a gastroenterologist if symptoms persist. If a thrombosed hemorrhoid is present and is painful, the patient should be referred to a surgeon.

Eating disorders

The physical examination of a patient with anorexia nervosa may reveal emaciation, dry skin, muscle wasting, peripheral edema, bradycardia, arrhythmias, hypotension, delayed sexual maturation, and stress fractures. A patient with bulimia nervosa may show erosion of the tooth enamel due to gastric-acid exposure, trauma to the hard or soft palate due to the insertion of fingers to induce vomiting, and cardiac arrhythmias if ipecac is used. The differential diagnosis includes gastrointestinal disorders, malignancies, depression, and psychiatric disorders. Tests that may be considered include CBC, BUN, lipid panel, LFTs, electrolytes, and electrocardiography. Management includes referral to a dietitian, a mental health counselor, and a family therapist. The patient should be hospitalized if weight is less than 70% of ideal body weight, if the patient is suicidal, or if outpatient treatment fails.

Two types of eating disorders are recognized:

- Anorexia nervosa: DSM-5 criteria include refusal to maintain normal body weight, fear of gaining weight even if underweight, disturbed body self-image, and amenorrhea on three consecutive cycles.
- Bulimia nervosa: DSM-5 criteria include recurrent episodes of binge eating followed by self-induced vomiting, misuse of laxatives, excessive exercise, or strict dieting at least twice weekly for at least three months along with excessive concern about body shape and weight.

Signs and symptoms of anorexia nervosa include fatigue, cold intolerance, muscle weakness, dizziness, fainting spells, amenorrhea, depression, compulsive exercising, and social isolation. Signs and symptoms of bulimia nervosa include menstrual irregularities, depression, anxiety, lack of meaningful relationships, impulsive behavior, and requests for diet pills or laxatives.

Cholecystitis

Cholecystitis, inflammation of the gall bladder, can result in obstruction of the bile duct related to calculi as well as pancreatitis from obstruction of the pancreatic duct. The disease is most common in overweight women ages 20 to 40, but it can occur in pregnant women and people of all ages, especially those who are diabetic or elderly. Children may develop cholecystitis secondary to cystic fibrosis, obesity, or total parenteral nutrition. Diagnosis is confirmed by ultrasound, as laboratory findings may be within the normal range.

Signs and symptoms include:

- Symptoms range from asymptomatic to severe right upper quadrant or epigastric pain, persisting two to six hours per episode.
- Disease of the biliary tract may cause radiation of pain to the back and nausea and vomiting.
- Cholangitis may result in jaundice and altered mental status.

Treatment includes:

- Antibiotics for sepsis or ascending cholangitis.
- Antispasmodic agents (glycopyrrolate) for biliary colic and vomiting.
- Analgesics (meperidine for acute pain).
- Antiemetics (promethazine).
- Laparoscopic or open cholecystectomy if warranted.

Appendicitis

Appendicitis is inflammation of the appendix that can lead to rupture and subsequent peritonitis. Signs and symptoms include periumbilical pain localizing to the RLQ over time. Associated symptoms may include anorexia, nausea, vomiting, fever, and diarrhea. Physical examination may reveal a low-grade fever, tenderness in the RLQ (McBurney's point), decreased bowel sounds, pain with flexion of hip against resistance (positive psoas sign), and painful RLQ when LLQ is palpated (Rosving's sign). The differential diagnosis includes ovarian cyst, ovarian torsion, ectopic pregnancy, pelvic inflammatory disease (PID), renal calculi, and cholecystitis. Tests that should be considered are WBC count, urinalysis, βHCG test, ultrasonography, and computerized tomography (CT). CT is generally not recommended for children or pregnant women to avoid ionizing radiation. The management of appendicitis is surgery.

Cystitis

Urinary infection, cystitis, is common and often-chronic low-grade kidney infections that develop over time. The most common cause is the bacteria *Escherichia coli*, part of the natural flora of the intestine. Women may develop infection after sexual intercourse.

Symptoms include:

- Changes in character of urine:
  - Appearance: The urine may become cloudy from mucus or purulent material. Hematuria may be present.
  - Color: Urine usually becomes concentrated and may be dark yellow/orange or brownish in color.
  - Odor: Urine may have a very strong or foul odor.
  - Output: Urinary output may decrease markedly.

- Pain: Suprapubic discomfort.
- Urgency, frequency.
- Systemic: Fever, chills, headache, and general malaise often accompany urine infections.

Treatment includes:

- Increased fluid intake.
- Antibiotics for 1 to 3 days: Trimethoprim-sulfa methoxazole, fluoroquinolones, or nitrofurantoin.
- Phenazopyridine 200 mg 3 times daily to relieve discomfort.
- Prophylactic antibiotic therapy: For females who have >3 episodes yearly.

Urethritis

Urethritis is inflammation of the urethra and can be caused by a variety of bacteria and viruses, especially those related to UTIs and STDs. Urethritis may also result from trauma or allergic sensitivity (such as to spermicides). Typical symptoms are similar to cystitis and can include burning, itching, urinary frequency and urgency, fever, and abdominal pain. Diagnostic procedures include pregnancy test, urinalysis and cultures, ultrasound, CBC, and C-reactive protein to determine the underlying cause. Treatment depends on the cause, but bacterial infections, such as *E. coli*, gonorrhea, and chlamydia are treated with antibiotics. If infection persists >6 weeks (chronic urethritis), a different type of antibiotic may be necessary. Uncontrolled infection may result in PID, cystitis, or cervicitis. Risk factors include high-risk sexual behavior, multiple sexual partners, poor hygiene, and history of STDs.

Hematuria

Most incidences of hematuria are relatively benign, such as hematuria caused by exercise, but hematuria should always be evaluated to determine if there is an underlying cause. Hematuria may be gross (obvious) or occult, found on examination. Bleeding sites may occur anywhere within the urinary tract. Common causes of hematuria include:

- Medications: ASA, warfarin, heparin, and clopidogrel.
- Cystitis and urethritis (especially in males): Urgency, frequency, burning.
- Renal infection: Flank pain, fever, chills.
- Renal/urinary calculi: Severe radiating pain in flank and/or abdomen.
- Cancer: Symptoms vary depending on location.
- Trauma: Ecchymosis, tenderness, guarding.

Diagnostic procedures may include UA with culture and sensitivities, renal function tests, cystoscopy, and CT scan (usually done now instead of IVP). Treatment depends on underlying cause, such as antibiotics for infection and fluids, analgesics, and ketorolac for small renal calculi or lithotripsy for larger calculi.

Renal and ureteral calculi

Renal and urinary calculi occur frequently, more commonly in males, and can relate to diseases (hyperparathyroidism, renal tubular acidosis, gout) and lifestyle factors, such as sedentary work. Additionally, some medications can precipitate calculi. Calculi can form at any age, most composed of calcium, and can range in size from very tiny to >6mm. Those <4mm can usually pass in the urine easily. Diagnostic studies include clinical findings, urinalysis (UA), pregnancy test to rule out ectopic pregnancy, BUN and creatinine if indicated, ultrasound (for pregnant women and children), and IV urography. Helical CT (noncontrast) is diagnostic. Symptoms occur with obstruction and are usually of sudden onset and acute:

- Severe flank pain radiating to the abdomen and ipsilateral testicle or labium majus.
- Nausea and vomiting.
- Diaphoresis.
- Hematuria.

Treatment includes:

- Analgesia: opiates and NSAIDs.
- Instructions and equipment for straining urine.
- Antibiotics if concurrent infection.
- Extracorporeal shock-wave lithotripsy.
- Surgical removal: percutaneous/standard nephrolithotomy.

Low back pain

Low back pain is a common in people engaged in strenuous exercise or work, especially heavy lifting. The spine comprises 24 vertebrae, which protect the spinal cord. Between the vertebrae are gelatinous intervertebral disks that serve as cushions. With injury, the intervertebral disk may herniate, bulge, or even rupture, causing pressure on the nerves. The most common injuries involve L4 to L5 and L5 to S1. Symptoms may vary but usually include sharp pain that radiates down the sciatic nerve in one or both legs and stiffness upon arising. Assessment should include type, intensity, site, and duration of pain as well as contributing factors (such as position). Range of motion and gait must be assessed. With disk herniation or injury to ligaments, flexion usually increases pain. Complete sensory and motor evaluation should be completed and the person referred for neurological care if there is any indication of serious injury. Treatment may include initial bed rest for one to two days followed by ambulation but restricted sitting until pain reduces. Pain medications, muscle relaxants, and hot and/or cold packs may relieve discomfort.

Strains

A strain is an overstretching of a part of the musculature ("pulled muscle") that causes microscopic tears in the muscle or tendon, usually resulting from excess stress, overuse of the muscle, blunt trauma, or overstretching. Common sites for strains include the ankle, back, and hamstrings. Onset of pain is usually sudden with local tenderness on use of the muscle. Strains are classified according to severity:

- First degree: This injury is relatively mild and symptoms, such as slight discomfort and tenderness to palpation, and it may be delayed until the following day.
- Second degree: Pain is usually felt on injury with tenderness on palpation and decreased passive and active range of motion, depending upon the site of injury. There may be signs of injury, such as edema and bruising.
- Third degree: The muscle or tendon is completely ruptured and pain occurs with injury. A defect may be palpable. Often there is extensive edema and bruising from injury to vasculature. Strength and loss of range of motion vary according to site of injury.

Sprains

A sprain is damage to a joint, with a partial rupture of the supporting ligaments, usually caused by wrenching or twisting that may occur with a fall. The rupture can damage blood vessels, resulting in edema, tenderness at the joint, and pain on movement with pain increasing over two to three hours after injury. An avulsion fracture (bone fragment pulled away by a ligament) may occur with strain, so x-rays rule out fractures. Sprains may be classified according to severity:

- First degree: This is a relatively mild degree of injury, usually associated with good range of motion and mild pain. Swelling may vary considerably, depending upon whether vessels are disrupted by the sprain.
- Second degree: This comprises a wide range of signs and symptoms, as there is further injury and partial rupture of the ligaments. Usually range of motion is limited by pain. Edema and bruising are usually present but vary in degree. The joint may be somewhat unstable.
- Third degree: This involves total rupture of the ligament with immediate marked pain (although sometimes less than with second degree), bruising, edema, and decreased range of motion. The joint is usually markedly unstable.

Seizure disorder

Seizure disorder is defined as the abnormal discharge of the neurons in the brain, which leads to changes in the functions of the body. Seizures are classified as follows:

- Partial: occur within a localized region of the brain
  - Simple partial: fully conscious
  - Complex partial: consciousness impaired
- Generalized : occur on both sides of the brain
  - Tonic-clonic ("grand mal")
  - Absence ("petit mal")
  - Myoclonic
  - Atonic ("drop seizures")

Causes of seizures include hypoxia, hypoglycemia, infection, fever, drug or medication toxicity, head injury, brain tumor, or CVA. Tests to be ordered include measurements of electrolytes, glucose, and BUN; LFTs; toxicology screening; and CBC. Procedures may include lumbar puncture, brain CT or MRI, and EEG. Management includes phenytoin (Dilantin), carbamazepine (Tegretol), valproic acid (Depakene), and clonazepam (Klonopin). All patients with first-time seizures or uncontrollable seizures should be referred to a neurologist.

Major depressive episode

A major depressive episode is a depressed mood, profound and constant sense of hopelessness and despair, or loss of interest in all or almost all activities for a period of at least two weeks. Family history of depression is a major risk factor. Developmental hormone changes at puberty or hormone disruption from disease can also contribute to depression. Depression is associated with neurotransmitter dysregulation, especially serotonin and norepinephrine. Major depression can be mild, moderate, or severe. Criteria include at least five of the following (including the first two):

- Depressed mood most of the day.
- Diminished interest in most or all activities previously found enjoyable.

- Significant weight gain or loss without dieting.
- Insomnia or hypersomnia.
- Persistent pessimism.
- Constant fatigue.
- Feelings of worthlessness.
- Reduced ability to focus on tasks.
- Recurring thoughts of death or suicide.

Treatment includes antidepressants, such as SSRIs, and cognitive behavioral therapy.

GAD

Generalized anxiety disorder (GAD) is an unrealistic apprehension and worry that persists for six or more months. GAD may be accompanied by tension, sweating, irritability, and hypervigilance. GAD is most common after age 20. Symptoms include:

- Motor tension: Tremulousness, muscle tension.
- Autonomic arousal: Shortness of breath, tachycardia, dry mouth, and diarrhea.
- Vigilance: Insomnia or other sleep disturbance and a feeling of being edgy.
- Depression.
- Impaired quality of life.

Levels of anxiety include:

- Mild: Slight physical arousal but retains the ability to learn well.
- Moderate: Physical symptoms are present.
- Severe: Physical symptoms interfere with day-to-day activities, difficulty concentrating, very anxious.
- Panic: Terrified, little or no ability to concentrate, shortness of breath, palpitations, fear of dying.

Treatment includes antianxiety medications, cognitive-behavioral therapy, and relaxation techniques.

Panic disorder

Panic disorder is chronic, repeated, and unexpected panic attacks, with spells of overwhelming fear, apprehension, terror, and being in danger when there is no specific cause. Characteristics include:

- Panic attack often begins with rapidly increasing sense of tragedy, coupled with tachycardia, difficulty breathing, and diaphoresis.
- Episodes last from minutes to several hours and may include sense of unreality, detachment from oneself, fainting, vertigo, choking, and chest pain. Initial attacks usually occur in an anxiety-provoking situation, while successive attacks are spontaneous and unexpected.
- Those affected often report to an emergency department thinking that they may be having a heart attack or severe respiratory problems.
- Anticipatory anxiety may exist between attacks because of fear that another may occur without warning.
- Severity of attacks may range from minimal to severe with disabling symptoms.

Treatment includes cognitive behavioral therapy, psychodynamic psychotherapy, and medications, including SSRIs, SNRIs, TCAs, benzodiazepines, and MAOIs.

OCD

Obsessive-compulsive disorder (OCD) is a disorder in which patients are plagued by obsessions and/or compulsions that interfere with employment and social, interpersonal, and other daily activities and last more than one hour daily. Characteristics include:

- Obsessions are unwanted, repeated, and uncontrollable ideas, images or urges that come to mind involuntarily despite attempts to ignore or suppress them.
- Compulsions are repeated, unwanted patterns of behavior (impulses) to perform apparently irrational or useless acts that are often responses to obsessions and done to reduce stress. Examples include:
  - o Cleaning and washing repeatedly to remove perceived contamination.
  - o Repeated checking or counting.
  - o Arranging and rearranging items.

A sense of dread may develop if the compulsion is resisted, and some try to ignore or suppress thoughts/behaviors. Intervention usually is not sought until emotional and/or physical exhaustion occurs in either the client or a significant other. Treatment includes cognitive behavioral therapy and antidepressants, including clomipramine, fluvoxamine, fluoxetine, sertraline, and paroxetine.

Diabetes

Diabetes is defined as a group of diseases that result in hyperglycemia. There are four types of diabetes:

- Type 1: total lack of insulin
- Type 2: persistent fasting hyperglycemia with insulin available
- Gestational diabetes: hyperglycemia due to pregnancy
- Secondary diabetes: hyperglycemia due to pancreatic disease or due to drug use

Complications of diabetes include coronary artery disease, cerebrovascular disease, nephropathy, retinopathy, peripheral neuropathy, and erectile dysfunction. Signs and symptoms include the classic triad of polyuria, polydipsia, and polyphagia. Other symptoms may include weight loss, fatigue, recurrent vaginal candidiasis, and changes in vision. Physical examination may reveal slow healing of skin trauma or infections, ulceration of the skin (especially in the lower extremities), hair loss in the lower extremities, retinopathy, diminished peripheral pulses, and sensory loss.

According to the American Diabetes Association, the diagnosis of diabetes can be made by any of the following tests:

- Fasting plasma glucose concentration of 126 mg/dL or higher
- Nonfasting plasma glucose concentration of 200 mg/dL or higher with symptoms of diabetes
- Oral glucose tolerance test of more than 200 mg/dL in the two-hour sample

The ADA recommends screening patients for diabetes if they exhibit the following characteristics, even if they have no symptoms: older than 45 years, overweight with a BMI of 25 or more, family history of diabetes, history of gestational diabetes, hypertension, or HDL cholesterol concentration of 35 mg/dL or less and/or a triglyceride concentration of 250 mg/dL or more. Goals of management should be a serum glucose concentration between 90 and 130 mg/dL. Hemoglobin A1C (HA1C), which reflects the average glucose levels over the last three months, should be lower than 7. Other tests that should be considered are lipid profile, serum creatinine measurement, and urinalysis.

The management of a patient with diabetes is as follows:

- The goal of treatment is to keep the plasma glucose concentration as close to normal as possible.
- Nonpharmacological treatment of Type 1 and Type 2 diabetes includes home glucose monitoring, smoking cessation, weight loss, exercise, proper diet, and reducing the LDL concentration.
- Pharmacological management of Type 1 diabetes includes the use of insulin to achieve tight control of plasma glucose concentrations. Such therapy may include rapid-acting, short-acting, intermediate-acting, or long-acting insulin. Pharmacological management of Type 2 diabetes includes the use of oral hypoglycemic agents such as sulfonylureas (Glipizide, Glyburide), biguanides (Metformin), and thiazolidinediones (Rosiglitazone).
- Patient and family education includes teaching about the use of medications, insulin injection techniques, the chronicity of the disease, the importance of adherence in maintaining the proper glucose concentration, glucose monitoring, weight management, diet, exercise, foot care, dental care, and contraception.
- Referral to a registered dietitian is indicated.

Hyperthyroidism

Hyperthyroidism is an excess of circulating thyroid hormone. Hyperthyroidism may be caused by any of the following conditions:

- Grave's disease: an autoimmune condition caused by excess synthesis and secretion of thyroid hormone as the result of circulating thyroid-stimulating immunoglobulins.
- Toxic multinodular goiter: accounts for most cases of hyperthyroidism in middle-aged and elderly patients
- Toxic adenoma: a single hyperfunctioning nodule encased in thyroid tissue
- Thyroiditis: a group of inflammatory conditions that cause excessive secretion of thyroid hormone

Signs and symptoms include increased appetite but weight loss, irritability, jitteriness, heat intolerance, sweating, fatigue, palpitations, tremors, diarrhea, and vision changes. Physical examination may reveal an enlarged or nodular thyroid gland, goiter, hyperreflexia, tremors, tachycardia, eyelid retraction secondary to exophthalmos, and increased bowel sounds.

Diagnostic tests that may be considered are TSH, radioactive iodine scan of the thyroid, and ultrasonography of the thyroid. Nonpharmacological management includes a proper diet and elimination of stimulants, such as caffeine and certain over-the-counter "cold" medications such as pseudoephedrine. Pharmacological management includes antithyroid drugs such as propylthiouracil (PTU) or methimazole (Tapazole), and radioactive iodine ablation (RIA). These drugs and procedures are contraindicated for pregnant or lactating women. Beta-blockers, such as atenolol and propanolol, may be given to slow heart rate and to provide general symptomatic relief. A low-dose sleeping medication may be needed until the thyroid hormone levels have decreased. Patient education includes teaching about on thyroid storm, which needs immediate attention. The patient may be referred to an endocrinologist, an ophthalmologist, a surgeon, and a dietitian.

Hypothyroidism

Hypothyroidism is defined as a deficiency of circulating thyroid hormone due to the failure of the thyroid to generate appropriate levels of thyroid hormone. Primary thyroid failure may be due to Hashimoto's thyroiditis, previous radioactive iodine treatment, or surgical removal of the gland. Secondary failure may be due to pituitary or hypothalamic disease. Risk factors include age older than 50 years, a history of autoimmune disease, and a family history of the disorder. Signs and symptoms may include weakness, dry skin, slow speech, forgetfulness, depression, cold intolerance, facial edema, constipation, and irregular menses. Physical examination may reveal an atrophic or goitrous thyroid gland, diminished reflexes, hearing loss, dry or coarse skin, bradycardia, anemia, and decreased bowel sounds.

Diagnostic testing may include TSH (which will be high in primary hypothyroidism but low in secondary hypothyroidism) and measurement of antimicrosomal antibodies, antithyroid peroxidases, and antithyroglobulin to determine Hashimoto's thyroiditis. Nonpharmacological management includes calorie restriction to prevent weight gain, a high-fiber and low-fat diet, smoking cessation, and exercise as tolerated. Pharmacological management includes the use of synthetic hormones such as levothyroxine sodium (Levoxyl, Synthroid). These must be prescribed as a low initial dosage that is slowly increased. Dosing too much too soon may put the patient into an iatrogenic hyperthyroid state. Referral to an endocrinologist is warranted if symptoms do not respond.

Anemia

Anemia is defined as an abnormally low hemoglobin concentration (<12 g/dL for women, <13 g/dL for men). Anemia is usually classified according to the mean corpuscular volume (MCV) of the RBC:

- Microcytic anemia: MCV <80 fL.* Examples are iron deficiency anemia and thalassemia trait.
- Macrocytic anemia: MCV >100 fL. Examples are B_{12} deficiency and folate deficiency.
- Normocytic anemia: MCV 80-100 fL. Examples are anemia of chronic disease, sickle cell disease, and renal failure.   *fL: femtoliters

Anemia may be asymptomatic, but signs and symptoms may also include fatigue, general weakness, dyspnea on exertion (DOE), headaches, and anorexia. Physical examination may reveal pallor of the skin or conjunctiva, glossitis, stomatitis, tachycardia, tachypnea, and thinning hair. Sickle cell crisis may include the above, along with elevated vital signs, hypotension, cyanosis, and scleral jaundice. Chronic sickle cell disease may present with cardiomegaly, skin ulcers (especially on lower extremities), osteomyelitis, retinopathy, and renal disease.

The management of the different types of anemias is as follows:

- Iron deficiency anemia (IDA): the source of the anemia needs to be found and corrected. Dietary iron intake should be increased, and the hemoglobin concentration should be checked regularly. Ferrous sulfate may be given for four to six months.
- Anemia of chronic disease: the only treatment for this anemia is treatment of the underlying disease.
- Vitamin B_{12} deficiency: B_{12} injections daily for 7 days, then weekly until hematocrit is normal, then monthly for life
- Folate deficiency: treatment includes increasing the dietary intake of legumes, leafy green vegetables, and liver. Folic acid supplements may be given.

- Sickle cell disease (SCD): all infections should be treated aggressively. Adequate hydration is essential. It is imperative that a patient with SCD receive annual pneumococcus and flu vaccinations.
- Refer the patient to a hematologist if resistant to treatment. Patient needs to go to the emergency department if sickle cell crisis occurs.

Thrombogenic disorders

Raynaud's disease

Raynaud's disease (RD) is a form of intermittent digital arteriolar vasoconstriction, especially in response to cold or stress. Primary RD occurs in 2 to 6% of the population, usually females, but RD can be secondary, primarily to rheumatic diseases. Secondary RD is usually more severe and may result in ulcerations or gangrene. Raynaud's phenomenon refers specifically to the vasoconstriction of arterioles of the hands and/or feet, resulting in pallor or cyanosis. A recovery phase results in hyperemia or rubor. Thus, symptoms are described as a progression from white to blue to red. The fingers are more often affected than the toes. Initially, just one or two fingertips are involved, but as the disease progresses, all the fingers to the distal palm are affected. Symptoms are bilateral with primary RD but may be unilateral with secondary RD. Symptoms may be triggered by exposure to cold, vasoconstrictive medications, and cigarette smoking. Treatment involves avoiding triggers, calcium channel blockers (nifedipine), or sympathectomy (for severe cases).

Polycythemia

Polycythemia is an increased volume of red blood cells (erythrocytes) >50% in females:

- Polycythemia vera is a proliferative disease in which myeloid cells overproduce blood cells, primarily red blood cells, although other cells and platelets are also elevated. The hematocrit may be >60%. Over time, the spleen enlarges and bone marrow becomes fibrotic, producing fewer cells. The disease may evolve into myeloid metaplasia with fibrosis or acute myelogenous leukemia. Patients are at increased risk of thrombosis because of increased viscosity of the blood. Treatment includes hydroxyurea to decrease production of RBCs, interferon to lower RBC counts, and scheduled phlebotomy to reduce RBC concentration. Hydration is especially important.
- Secondary polycythemia results from increased production of erythropoietin, which stimulates the bone marrow to produce more red blood cells. This may result from neoplasms (such as renal cell carcinoma), COPD, heart disease, or altitude sickness— conditions that cause hypoxia, which stimulates production of erythropoietin. Identifying the underlying cause is critical to treatment.

DIC

DIC (consumption coagulopathy) is a secondary disorder that is triggered by another, such as trauma, congenital heart disease, necrotizing enterocolitis, sepsis, and severe viral infections. DIC triggers both coagulation and hemorrhage. The onset of symptoms of DIC may be very rapid or a slower. Those who develop the chronic manifestation usually have fewer acute symptoms and may slowly develop ecchymosis, bleeding wounds, and/or blood clots.

Symptoms include:

- Bleeding from surgical or venous puncture sites.
- Evidence of GI bleeding with distention, bloody diarrhea.
- Hypotension and acute symptoms of shock.

- Petechiae and purpura with extensive bleeding into the tissues.
- Laboratory abnormalities:
  o Prolonged prothrombin and partial prothrombin times.
  o Decreased platelet counts and fragmented RBCs.
  o Decreased fibrinogen.

Treatment includes:

- Identifying and treating underlying cause.
- Replacement blood products, such as platelets and fresh frozen plasma.
- Anticoagulation therapy (heparin) to increase clotting time.
- Cryoprecipitate to increase fibrinogen levels.
- Coagulation inhibitors and coagulation factors.

APAS

Antiphospholipid antibody syndrome (APAS) is a primary autoimmune disorder characterized by recurrent venous or arterial occlusion (such as DVT and pulmonary embolism), recurrent miscarriage, or thrombocytopenia with presence of antiphospholipid antibodies (lupus anticoagulant, anticardiolipin, or beta-2 glycoprotein) but without other indications of systemic lupus erythematosus (SLE). A secondary form has similar symptoms but is related to the primary disease, such as SLE. Symptoms vary widely and may include those related to vascular occlusion (pain, swelling, circulatory impairment), headache, rash, mitral valve regurgitation, bleeding (ecchymosis, petechiae, choreiform movements, loss of hearing, and cognitive impairment. Risk factors include other autoimmune disorder, medications (hydralazine, phenytoin, and amoxicillin), infections (syphilis, HIV, HCV, and malaria), and genetic predisposition. Triggering factors can include pregnancy, surgery, oral contraceptives, smoking, hypertension, and extended immobility (sitting). Thrombosis may result in severe organ damage. Treatment first includes heparin to stabilize, then Warfarin, and sometimes low-dose aspirin. However, warfarin is contraindicated with pregnancy.

Anaphylaxis syndrome

Anaphylaxis syndrome is a sudden acute systemic immunoglobulin E (IgE) or nonimmunoglobulin E (non-IgE) inflammatory response affecting the cardiopulmonary and other systems.

- IgE-mediated response (anaphylactic shock) is an antibody–antigen reaction against an allergen, such as milk, peanuts, latex, insect bites, drugs, or fish. This is the most common type.
- Non IgE-mediated response (anaphylactoid reaction) is a systemic reaction to infection, exercise, radio contrast material or other triggers. While the response is almost identical to the other type, it does not involve IgE.

Typically, with IgE-mediated response, an antigen triggers release of substances, such as histamine and prostaglandins, which affect the skin and the cardiopulmonary and GI systems. Histamine causes initial erythema and edema by inducing vasodilation. Each time the person has contact with the antigen, more antibodies form in response, and allergic reactions worsen. Anaphylactic shock related to anesthesia is rare, although anaphylactoid reactions may occur with opioids, hypnotics, and muscle relaxants. Antibiotics (penicillin, sulfonamides, cephalosporins) and latex allergy cause most medication/treatment related anaphylaxis.

RA

Rheumatoid arthritis (RA) is an autoimmune disease characterized by erosive destruction of the synovial tissue of the joints. The exact etiology of RA is unknown. The American College of Rheumatology lists the following criteria for the diagnosis of RA:

- Morning stiffness and swelling of at least three joints lasting more than one hour
- Swelling of the proximal interphalangeal (PIP), metacarpophalangeal (MCP), or wrist joints
- Symmetrical joint swelling
- Subcutaneous nodules
- Positive rheumatoid factor (RF)
- Radiographic evidence of RA

Signs and symptoms may include morning joint stiffness lasting more than one hour, joint pain, joint swelling and redness, fatigue, depression, malaise, and low-grade fever. Physical examination may reveal symmetrical soft-tissue swelling over the PIP or MCP, deformity of the joints, limited range of motion, subcutaneous nodules, lymphadenopathy, splenomegaly, and ophthalmological symptoms. Test to be ordered include RF, ESR, and radiography of affected joints.

Nonpharmacological treatment may include smoking cessation, rest, and exercise as tolerated. Initial pharmacological management may include the use of NSAIDs to manage pain and inflammation. As the disease progresses, disease-modifying antirheumatic drugs (DMARDs) may be needed. These drugs include hydroxychloroquine (Plaquenil), sulfasalazine (Azulfidine), methotrexate (Rheumatrex), leflunomide (Avara), and infliximab (Remicade). Patient education should include safety to prevent injuries, discussion of tonicity and episodic nature of the problem, and the noncontagious nature of the disease. Referral to an RA support group may be helpful. Referral to several specialists, including a rheumatologist, a podiatrist, an orthopedist, and a physical therapist, may be warranted.

SLE

Systemic lupus erythematosus (SLE) is a chronic inflammatory disorder of the immune system; its symptoms wax and wane. The etiology of SLE is an abnormal response of the immune system, which creates antibodies to normal tissue. According to the American College of Rheumatology, four of the following 11 criteria must be present to verify the diagnosis of SLE:

- Malar rash
- Discoid rash
- Photosensitivity
- Oral lesions
- Arthritis involving two or more peripheral joints
- Pleuritis, pericarditis, or peritonitis
- Seizures or psychosis
- Hemolytic anemia, leucopenia, or thrombocytopenia
- Positive antineutrophil antibody (ANA) test
- False-positive syphilis serology
- Positive lupus erythematosus (LE) prep

Signs and symptoms may include fever, malaise, arthralgias, photosensitivity, headaches, depression, and seizures. Physical examination may reveal malar rash (a rash over the cheeks), discoid rash, alopecia, oral lesions, pleurisy, or pericarditis. Tests that may be considered include ANA, VDRL, LE prep, CBC, creatinine, and urinalysis.

Nonpharmacological treatment includes rest, avoidance of direct sunlight, proper diet, exercise, smoking cessation, and minimal alcohol intake. Pharmacological treatment includes the use of NSAIDs to control arthralgias and fever. Corticosteroids are used if life-threatening symptoms develop. Long-term therapy may include the use of hydroxychloroquine (Plaquenil), an antimalarial drug. Side effects may include retinopathy, corneal edema, rash, pruritus, and hematological problems. Patient education includes the use of sunscreens, avoidance of direct sunlight, relaxation, stress reduction, exercise, prompt treatment of any infections, avoidance of pregnancy, and avoidance of surgery or dental procedures during SLE flares. Immunizations should be up-to-date; however, it is not advisable to use live-virus vaccines if the patient has SLE. The patient should be referred to a rheumatologist. Social services should also be contacted if the disease is disabling.

HIV

Human immunodeficiency virus (HIV) is a virus that attacks the human immune system and results in a spectrum of symptoms ranging from no symptoms at all to immunosuppression resulting in acquired immune deficiency syndrome (AIDS). The HIV virus is transmitted through contact with an infected person's blood, blood products, semen, vaginal secretions, or other bodily fluids. Risk factors include unprotected sex, multiple sexual partners, intravenous drug use, birth of an infant to an infected mother, blood transfusion, and organ transplant. Signs and symptoms initially include flu-like symptoms, fever, diarrhea, joint pain, and oral lesions. As seroconversion progresses, the immune system starts to weaken (may take eight to twelve years), and symptoms of fatigue, headache, arthralgia, weight loss, night sweats, chills, and opportunistic infections begin. As the disease evolves into AIDS, severe infections occur as the immune system is further damaged.

The following are physical examination findings and the tests that should be ordered for a patient with HIV infection:

- Findings of advancing HIV/AIDS may include the following: oral, vaginal, penile, or skin *Candida* infections; toxoplasmosis; malignancies; Kaposi's sarcoma; lymphoma; squamous cell carcinoma; and tuberculosis. The main defining diagnosis of AIDS is *Pneumocystis carinii* pneumonia.
- Tests that may be considered include enzyme-linked immunosorbent assay (ELISA), the results of which will be positive if HIV antibodies are present, and Western Blot to verify ELISA. For HIV-positive women, screening tests should include CBC every three months, chemistry panel every six months, RPR or VDRL every 6 to 12 months, baseline tests for hepatitis A, B and C, chest radiography, PPD every six months, and Pap test every six months.
- The CD4+ cell count should be measured every three months. The normal range is $800/mm^3$ to $1,050/mm^3$; when the count drops below $200 /mm^3$, the patient is likely to have symptoms of AIDS.

The management of a patient with HIV infection/AIDS is as follows:

- Antiviral therapy includes highly active antiretroviral therapy (HAART), which combines three or four drugs to suppress the virus. The goal is to reduce the HIV RNA concentration to below 500 copies/mL for as long as possible; however, because HIV mutates rapidly, treatment may have to be changed periodically.

- Drugs that are used are called antiretroviral drugs; these drugs include nucleoside reverse transcriptase inhibitors (NRTIs), nonnucleoside reverse transcriptase inhibitors (NNRTIs), and protease inhibitors (PIs).
- Patient education includes teaching patients not to breastfeed, to practice safe sex, not to share needles, to stop smoking, to stop using street drugs, to decrease alcohol intake, to eat a healthy diet, to exercise, and to avoid exposure to pets.
- Any patient who tests positive for the HIV virus should be referred to an infectious disease specialist.

Breast screening

Below are the criteria recommended by the American Cancer Society and the National Cancer Institute for screening mammography and the limitations of mammography:

- Women aged 40 to 50 years:
  - The American Cancer Society (ACS) recommends screening mammography annually.
  - The National Cancer Institute (NCI) recommends screening mammography every one to two years.
- For women aged 50 years or older, annual screening is recommended.
- The breast tissue of younger women is denser than that of older patients; therefore, screening mammography is less reliable for younger women.
- The false-negative rate for screening mammography ranges from 10% to 15%.
- Screening mammography is less accurate for women with breast implants than for women without augmentation; however, the false-positive rate is not higher.
- If a woman has a strong family history of breast masses or breast cancer (for example, breast cancer in her mother or sister), more frequent screening may be warranted.

Colorectal screening

Recommendations for colorectal screening are based on age and risk:

- Age 50—Average risk: Asymptomatic without risk factors.
- Age 40—Increased risk:
  - Family history of colorectal cancer in first- or second-degree relatives.
  - Family history of genetic syndrome (FAP, HNLPCC).
  - Adenomatous polyps in first-degree relatives before age 60.
  - History of polyps or colorectal cancer, history of inflammatory bowel disease.

Fecal occult blood	**Yearly: checks for blood in stool.**
Flexible sigmoidoscopy	**Every 5 years**: scope to check for polyps or signs of cancer in rectum and lower third of colon. (Often done with fecal occult blood test.)
Colonoscopy	**Every 10 years** or as a follow-up for abnormalities in other screening: longer flexible scope, usually with anesthesia, to check the rectum and the entire colon. It allows for removal of polyps, small cancerous lesions, and biopsies and provides surveillance of inflammatory bowel disease.
Double contrast barium enema	**Every 5 years**: x-ray with contrast to visualize intestinal abnormalities.

Endometrial cancer screening

Screening for endometrial cancer may be done if a Pap smear is positive or if risk factors for uterine cancer are present, including early menarche, late menopause, nulliparity, Polycystic ovary syndrome (*PCOS*), history of breast or ovarian cancer, obesity, history of pelvic radiation, and family history of uterine cancer. Women should be informed of risks and symptoms related to endometrial cancer and should note any sign of spotting or vaginal bleeding. Endometrial cancer usually causes bleeding, so most cancers are diagnosed early. Those with risk factors or suspected cancer should be examined. Tests used for screening include:

- Pap smear: May show abnormal endometrial cells incidentally but is not intended for endometrial screening.
- Transvaginal ultrasound (TVU): Indicated for those with or at risk for hereditary nonpolyposis colon cancer annually and for those with abnormal vaginal bleeding.
- Endometrial biopsy: Indicated for abnormal vaginal bleeding.

Screening guidelines have not been established for endometrial cancer, and routine TUV and endometrial biopsies do not appear to improve outcomes.

Lung cancer screening

Routine screening for lung cancer in the absence of symptoms is not recommended because chest x-rays and sputum cytology have not proven effective at early diagnosis, and repeated exposure to radiation increases risk of cancer. Patients with risk factors should be educated about possible symptoms.

Risk factors include:

- Any history of smoking (cigarettes, marijuana, crack cocaine).
- Exposure to second-hand smoke.
- Exposure to environmental toxins (asbestos, radon, chemicals).
- Family history of lung or GU cancer.

Symptoms include:

- Hemoptysis.
- Dyspnea.
- Persistent cough.
- Recurrent bronchitis/pneumonia.
- Clubbing.

If symptoms occur, screening tests may include spirometry, chest x-ray, and spiral CT scan (which is most effective at identifying small lesions). CT scan cannot differentiate cancer from other lesions, such as scar tissue or infection, so when small lesions are evident, a course of antibiotics may be given to determine if the lesions resolve. Repeat CT may be done to determine if lesion is growing (an indication of cancer). Screening recommendations have not yet been established, although clinical trials are in progress to determine the efficacy of different protocols.

Skin cancer screening

Routine screening for skin cancer is not recommended for all adults, although yearly dermatological examination is recommended for those at risk for skin cancer because of personal history of melanoma or other malignant skin cancer. Other risk factors for which the person should receive an assessment and possible follow-up routine examinations include:

- Family history of melanoma (≥ relatives).
- Presence of actinic keratoses.
- Presence of multiple and/or atypical nevi.

Additionally, all patients should be advised to use sunscreen and avoid excessive (≥ 20 minutes daily) exposure to direct sunlight. FDA guidelines advise that people should use sunscreen labeled "broad spectrum," which protects against both ultraviolet A (UVA) and ultraviolet B (UBV) rays. Effective sunscreen must have a sun protection factor (SPF) of ≥ 15. Sunscreen should be reapplied every 2 hours. Water-resistant (swimming, perspiring) sunscreen must be reapplied every 40 to 80 minutes (specified on the label).

Cardiovascular screening

Cholesterol

The NIH, NHLBI Report of the National Cholesterol Education Program Expert Panel on Detection, Evaluation, and Treatment of High Blood Cholesterol in Adults stresses that LDL cholesterol is the major cause of coronary heart disease (CHD). The optimal LDL level is < 100 mg/dL. Management strategies include:

- Risk assessment: A fasting lipoprotein profile should be obtained for adults ≥ 20 every 5 years. Major risk factors that modify LDL goals include smoking, hypertension, HDL < 40 mg/dL, family history of premature CHD (or risk equivalent, such as diabetes, peripheral arterial disease, abdominal aortic aneurysm, and carotid arterial disease), and age ≥ 45 for men and ≥ 55 for women.
- Determining primary or secondary causes: If LDL is elevated, causes of secondary dyslipidemia should be assessed prior to treatment. Secondary causes include diabetes, hypothyroidism, obstructive liver disease, chronic kidney failure, and drugs (progestins, anabolic steroids, corticosteroids).

High blood pressure

The Seventh Report of the Joint National Committee on Prevention, Detection, Evaluation, and Treatment of High Blood Pressure makes a number of specific recommendations regarding evaluation:

- Follow-up: Recheck in 2 years for normal, 1 year for prehypertension, 2 months for stage 1 and 1 month for stage 2. Immediate treatment for BP > 180/110 mm Hg.
- Ambulatory BP: Done for suspected white-coat (reactive) hypertension if no target damage to organs (heart, brain, chronic kidney disease, peripheral artery disease, or retinopathy), drug resistance, hypotension related to antihypertensives, episodic hypertension, and autonomic dysfunction.
- Diagnostic tests: 12-lead EKG, urinalysis, blood glucose, Hct, K, creatinine (with estimated glomerular filtration rate—GFR), calcium, lipoprotein profile.

Osteoporosis

Osteoporosis is defined as low bone density along with structural deterioration that leads to bone fragility and increased risk of fractures. Signs and symptoms include backache, collapse of vertebrae, and bones that easily fracture. Physical examination may reveal kyphosis and loss of

- 76 -

height due to collapsing vertebrae and unexpected fractures of the spine, hips, or wrists. Diagnostic tests may include bone mineral density (BMD), dual-energy x-ray absorptiometry (DEXA), single-energy x-ray absorptiometry (SXA), and quantitative ultrasound (QUS). Radiography is used mainly to detect osteoporotic fractures. Laboratory tests used to rule out secondary causes of osteoporosis include parathyroid hormone (PTH) level, TSN, dexamethasone suppression test, and measurement of urine cortisol level.

Nonpharmacological management includes adequate intake of dietary calcium and vitamin D. Resistance (weight-bearing) exercises three times per week will help mobilize the calcium to move into the bones, thereby strengthening them. Aerobic exercise, such as walking, running, or swimming three times per week will help keep ligaments, tendons, and muscles toned. Exercise will also help maintain proprioception, thereby helping to prevent falls. Smoking cessation and alcohol intake minimization should be recommended. Pharmacological management includes the use of oral bisphosphonates such as alendronate (Fosamax) or risedronate (Actonel), which inhibit the resorption of bone. Hormones that inhibit bone resorption of calcium, such as calcitonin-salmon (Fortical, Miacalcin) nasal spray, may also be prescribed.

Diet and nutrition

According to *Dietary Guidelines for Americans, 2010*, people should maintain a balanced caloric intake and eat more nutrient-dense foods and fluids. Diet and nutrition recommendations include:

Sodium: < 2300 mg/day and 1500 mg/day for those ≥ 51 years or African American or with existing cardiovascular or renal disease or diabetes. Saturated fat: < 10% of calories. Dietary cholesterol: < 300 mg/day. Alcohol: ≤ 1 drink daily for women and ≤2 for men.	Fruits Grains Dairy Vegetables Protein	Eat more fruits and dark green, red, and orange vegetables. Replace half of refined grains with whole grain. Use lower fat milk products. Eat a variety of high-protein foods, including seafood, beans, and nuts. Replace solid fats with oils. Limit trans fatty acids, solid fats, sugar, and refined grains.

Pregnant women are advised to choose foods high in heme iron and vitamin C and take 400 mcg of synthetic folic acid daily. Breastfeeding women should eat 8 to 12 ounces of seafood per week but limit white tuna to 6 ounces and avoid tilefish, shark, swordfish, and king mackerel. People > 50 should include food or supplements with vitamin B12.

Weight loss medications

Several weight management medications are approved by the FDA:

- Orlistat (Xenical©): A lipase inhibitor, orlistat blocks the enzyme lipase, which is responsible for breaking down fat. Adverse effects of this medication include loose stools, flatulence, and abdominal cramping.
- Sibutramine (Meridia©): Sibutramine is an appetite suppressant. Adverse effects include elevated blood pressure, dry mouth, tachycardia, headache, and constipation. Insomnia can occur if the medication is taken late in the day

- Phentermine: Phentermine is an appetite suppressant available in three dosage strengths. The lowest dose should always be used first, because tolerance develops rapidly. Adverse effects of phentermine are tachycardia, dry mouth, and constipation. Insomnia can occur if the medication is taken late in the day. Of the three most popular weight management medications, phentermine is the least expensive.

Follow up for obese patient

The following are appropriate methods of follow-up for an obese patient:

- Prescribe only a 30-day supply of medication with no refills. This will encourage your patient to return each month so that you can monitor her weight and answer her questions. She should understand that medication is a temporary measure.
- Pay particular attention to blood pressure and pulse rate during each visit. Sibutramine and phentermine can increase blood pressure.
- Discuss the patient's exercise status. Reinforce the concept of resistance training; she needs to increase her muscle mass to minimize the flabbiness associated with weight loss.
- Congratulate the patient for positive fat loss to encourage her to continue.
- Advise her that her weight or fat loss may plateau periodically as her body adjusts to her new body fat level. Tell her to not be discouraged and to continue her exercise regimen.
- Follow up every thirty days.

Example weight loss management

The management of a woman who requests help in losing weight, whose vital signs are normal, and whose BMI is 29 is as follows:

- Determine whether there is any organic reason for her overweight
- If the findings of physical examination are normal, prescribe an exercise program involving walking one-half hour each day
- Recommend that the patient keep a food diary
- Order laboratory tests: measurements of thyroid stimulating hormone (TSH), glucose and HA1C, and βHCG, and a lipid panel

Smoking cessation

The U.S. Department of Health and Human Services guidelines for helping smokers quit include:

- Ask about and record smoking status at every visit.
- Advise all smokers to quit and explain health reasons.
- Assess readiness to quit by questioning and if willing, provide resources. If the patient is not willing, provide support and attempt to motivate the person to quit with information.
- Assist smokers with a plan that sets a date (within two weeks), removes cigarettes, enlists family and friends, reviews past attempts, and anticipates challenges during the withdrawal period. The nurse practitioner must give advice about the need for abstinence and discuss the association of smoking with drinking. Medications to help control the urge to smoke (patches, gum, lozenge, prescriptions) and resources should be provided.
- Do follow-up monitoring to evaluate progress and reinforce the program.

Aging

Older adults face many changes associated with aging, such as social isolation, stress, loss, and health issues. As people age, they need to take active steps to deal with aging and prevent complications:

- Diet: The need for vitamin B12 increases with age, and because obesity is an increasing problem and a cause of morbidity in older adults, some modifications in diet (lowered calories, increased nutrition) may be necessary. Referral to a dietitian for meal planning may benefit some adults.
- Exercise: Older adults should strive to exercise at least 30 minutes daily for ≥5 days weekly. Endurance, strengthening, stretching, and balance exercises are recommended if physical condition allows.
- Activity: Engaging with others helps to prevent social isolation. Older adults should consider senior citizens' groups, social networking sites or message boards, and other organizations.
- Routine health examinations, vaccinations, and screening: Early identification of disease and treatment can prevent much morbidity associated with chronic conditions. Vaccinations should include annual influenza and herpes zoster (shingles). Smoking cessation and moderate drinking are advised.

Parenting

Most mothers benefit from information about parenting, especially new mothers, who may have little experience caring for children or know little about child development. Information should include:

- Information resources: Pamphlets, books, videos, the Internet, community agencies, and libraries.
- Childcare options: Babysitters, childcare centers, and cooperatives.
- Behavioral management: Age-appropriate expectation, rules, consequences (negative and positive), modeling appropriate behavior, role-playing, dealing with challenges, toilet training, and effective praising.
- Discipline: Behavior modification, consequences, scolding, time-out, and reasoning.
- Bonding: Physical contact, reading, holding, talking, and making time.

Most mothers benefit from information about parenting, especially new mothers, who may have little experience caring for children or know little about child development. Information should include:

- Parenting styles: Indifferent (shows little warmth, neglectful), permissive (shows warmth but no rules or guidance), authoritarian (shows little warmth, communicates little, inflexible), and authoritative (shows warmth, provides guidance with minimal restraints, communicates, is flexible). (Authoritative is preferred.)
- Community resources: Playgroups, WIC program, Head Start, and Child Protective Services.
- Nutrition: Breastfeeding, bottle-feeding, introduction of food, and age-appropriate diets.
- Common health problems: Colic, upper respiratory infections, diaper rash, diarrhea, and constipation.

Prevention of sexually transmitted diseases

The CDC has developed five strategies to prevent and control the spread of sexually transmitted diseases:

- Educate those at risk about how to make changes in sexual practices to prevent infection.
- Identify symptomatic and asymptomatic infected persons who may not seek diagnosis or treatment.
- Diagnose and treat those who are infected.
- Prevent infection of sex partners through evaluation, treatment, and counseling.
- Provide preexposure vaccination for those at risk.

Practitioners are advised to take sexual histories of patients and to assess risk. The 5-P approach to questioning is advocated. One should ask about:

- Partners: Gender and number.
- Pregnancy prevention: Birth control.
- Protection: Methods used.
- Practices: Type of sexual practices (oral, anal, vaginal) and use of condoms.
- Past history of STDs: High-risk behavior (promiscuity, prostitution) and disease risk (HIV/hepatitis).

The CDC recommends a number of specific preventive methods as part of the clinical guidelines for prevention of sexually transmitted diseases:

- Abstinence/reduction in the number of sex partners.
- Preexposure vaccination: All those evaluated for STD should receive the hepatitis B vaccination, and men who have sex with men (MSM) and illicit drug users should receive hepatitis A vaccination.
- Male latex (or polyurethane) condoms should be used for all sexual encounters with only water-based lubricants used with latex.
- Female condoms may be used if male condom can't be used properly.
- Condoms and diaphragms should not be used with spermicides containing nonoxynol-9 (N-9), and N-9 should not be used as a lubricant for anal sex.
- Nonbarrier contraceptive measures provide no protection from STDs and must not be relied on to prevent disease.
- Women should be counseled regarding emergency contraception with medication or insertion of a copper IUD.

Stress management

While it's not possible to eliminate all stress, people can learn to manage stress so it has less emotional and physical impact on their lives. Stress management techniques include:

- Relaxation exercises:
  - Meditation/breathing exercises: Slow in and out breaths while repeating a word or phrase.
  - Massage: Self-massage or massage by others.
  - Progressive relaxation techniques.

- Visualization exercises/Positive thinking: Use the power of the mind to imagine a more positive outcome.
- Time management: Establish priorities, make a schedule, and delegate.
- Exercise: Increase activity and exercise 20 to 30 minutes daily.
- Breaks: Plan regular breaks from work or other activities, 5 to 15 minutes.
- Snacks: Prepare healthy snacks and avoid high-sugar/high-fat snack foods.
- Hobbies or interests: Find an outlet, such as reading, music, painting, or crafts.

Laboratory tests for fatigue

The following are the laboratory tests that should be ordered for a patient reporting fatigue and the rationale for ordering each test:

- CBC: This test can determine whether the patient is anemic. A low red blood cell (RBC) count can cause fatigue because there are fewer RBCs to carry oxygen to the tissues. A very high white blood cell (WBC) count can imply infection or malignancy.
- Thyroid function tests: Hypothyroidism can cause chronic fatigue.
- Glucose concentration and HA1C: A high serum glucose concentration and an elevated HA1C imply diabetes, a common cause of fatigue.
- βHCG: Pregnant women commonly experience fatigue.
- ESR/ANA: Fatigue is a primary symptom of systemic lupus erythematosus, an autoimmune disease of generally unknown origin.
- LFTs: Hepatic disease, such as hepatitis, can cause fatigue.
- BUN/creatinine concentration: Elevation of the BUN or creatinine concentrations suggests a buildup of waste products in the body, which can lead to fatigue.

Partner/spousal abuse

Abuse is defined as physical, emotional, or sexual mistreatment or violence. More than half of all women experience some form of abuse during their lifetimes. Examples of abuse are as follows:

- Physical abuse - Slapping; Punching; Pushing; Locking one out of house; Locking one in the house; Refusing to provide medical care; Refusing to buy food; Destroying personal property
- Emotional abuse - Name-calling; Making insulting remarks; Refusing visits to family or friends; Humiliating one in public; Withholding affection
- Sexual - Treating women as sexual objects; Forcing sexual acts; Withholding sex and affection as "punishment"; Performing sadistic sexual acts
- Diagnosis of abuse
- History - Depression; Suicide gestures; History of sexual or physical abuse as a child; Multiple injuries with no acceptable explanation; Repeated STDs; Repeated spontaneous abortions
- Physical examination- Assess injuries; Note delayed treatment of previous injuries; Note patterned injuries- Belt marks; Rope burns; Bite marks; Bruising consistent with grasping; Note physical findings that do not correlate with history; Note genital trauma

Genetics

Genetic counseling is usually triggered because a woman has concerns about genetic disease or because of maternal risk factors, such as age. Counseling is especially important because a number of ethical issues must be addressed with genetic testing, including diagnostic and predictive testing and options such as elective abortion. Genetic counseling should be nondirective in that it provides information and support while allowing the patient to make decisions free of the counselor's bias. Preconception counseling includes these different aspects:

- Medical: Includes information about possible diagnoses and risks to the fetus and mother.
- Informative: Educates patient (and partner) about the genetic condition, course of the disease, patterns of inheritance, risks for future pregnancies, testing availability, and treatment options.
- Supportive: Provides emotional support and assists patient (and partner) to locate other sources of support, such as support groups, national organizations, Internet blogs and message boards, as well as psychosocial and religious organizations.

Environment

Preconception counseling should include an assessment of environmental concerns:

- Lead: Lead-based paint was commonly used up until the 1970s, so older homes should be inspected for signs of peeling, chalky, or crumbling paint, which increases risk of lead poisoning. If necessary, lead paint should be removed by licensed contractors. Local water companies should have information about lead pipes and the danger of lead in water. Lead crystal glassware and some imported ceramic ware also pose risks. Solvents should be avoided or used with care and sufficient ventilation.
- Chemicals/metals: Workplace chemicals may pose risks during pregnancy, so OSHA guidelines must be followed to ensure safety. Dental offices and some industries may increase risk of mercury exposure. Women should prevent excessive mercury exposure by avoiding tilefish, shark, king mackerel, and swordfish and limiting albacore tuna to ≤ 6 ounces/week.
- Smoke/carbon monoxide: Smoke and carbon monoxide detectors must be in place. Mothers should not smoke and should avoid exposure to secondhand smoke.

Lifestyle

Lifestyle counseling recognizes that the traditional nuclear family is no longer the sole model for childrearing. Different lifestyles require adjustments in traditional roles:

- Dual career/dual earner: One parent may take family leave or parents make arrangements for childcare.
- Single parent: Single parents often face difficulties in trying to support and care for a child and may suffer economic hardship. Issues may include use of a sperm donor and paternal responsibility.
- Cohabiting: Unmarried heterosexual couples live together with some similarities to the nuclear family, but legal and financial responsibilities of a child must be decided.
- Gay/lesbian: Whether gays and lesbians marry or cohabit they create families in nontraditional ways. For example, lesbians may use sperm donors. Gay couples often adopt. Children in these families may face social pressures because of their parents' lifestyles, but these children tend to fare as well as those raised in heterosexual households.

Medications

Safe medications during pregnancy

Allergies	**Diphenhydramine or loratadine.**
Constipation	Fiber-based products, such as Metamucil. Stool softeners. Milk of magnesia (should use rarely).
Diarrhea	May use antidiarrheals, such as Kaopectate and Imodium after the first trimester.
Headache, pain	Acetaminophen
Heartburn	Products with aluminum, such as Maalox, Mylanta, and Gaviscon, can be used but should be limited. Calcium-based products, such as Tums, are a better choice.
Monilial infection	Miconazole or terconazole
Nausea and vomiting	Vitamin B6 (100 mg tab). Emetrol.
Skin rash	Topical hydrocortisone cream/ointment. Caladryl. Benadryl lotion/cream.
URIs	Acetaminophen, pseudoephedrine (Sudafed), Vicks cough syrup, Robitussin DM. Avoid cold preparations with sustained action or indications for multisymptoms.

Nutrition

Preconception nutrition

Weight management	Underweight is associated with LBW, and overweight is associated with increased complications.
Balanced diet	Guidelines for general nutrition should be followed, including adequate intake of protein, whole grains, fruits, vegetables, and dairy products. Insure adequate iron intake through diet (meats, poultry, fish, green leafy vegetables, legumes) and/or supplementation
Folic acid	400 mg daily through supplements as well as increased intake of berries, nuts, whole grains, and green leafy vegetables to decrease incidence of neural tube defects.
Calcium	≥ 1000 mcg/day through supplements or three glasses of skim milk daily.
Caffeine	Caffeine products (tea, coffee, and chocolate) should be decreased or eliminated, as studies have indicated that caffeine may reduce fertility.
Artificial sweeteners	Safe sweeteners include Stevia, aspartame (in limited amounts), and sucralose (Splenda). Avoid saccharine, as its safety is not clear.

Patient counseling and education topics

The following items should be discussed with the patient during the counseling and education period:

- Risky behaviors
- Nutrition
- Calcium
  - Aged 50-64, not taking estrogen: 1500 mg/day
  - Aged 50-64, taking estrogen: 1000 mg/day
  - Aged 65+: 1500 mg/day
- Factors that may interfere with calcium absorption
  - Soft drinks; Caffeine; High protein intake;
  - Tobacco products; Excessive alcohol intake
- Breast and skin examination, including use of mirror or partner to inspect back
- Genital examination, including use of mirror to inspect perineum and other genital areas not visually accessible
- Physical activity
  - 30+ minutes of aerobic exercise per day, such as walking, bike riding, or using a treadmill. Jogging may be encouraged if the patient is physically capable and if no other medical reasons preclude such exercise.
  - Resistance training (weight lifting) is imperative for maintaining and increasing bone density and muscle mass.
  - Daily stretching exercises will help maintain flexibility.
  - Exercise will help keep body fat under control and will decrease stress.

Gynecology

Female breast

The anatomy of the female breast is as follows:

- Breast: modified sweat glands that produce milk in the female
- Lobes: approximately 15 to 20 per breast, extending to the upper outer quadrant of each breast and ending in the tail of Spencer, which terminates in the axilla
- Lobules: branches of lobes that contain lactiferous sinuses that direct milk toward the nipple
- Alveoli: responsible for the production of milk; located at the ends of the lobules
- Nipple: composed of erectile tissue at which the lactiferous sinuses terminate and where milk secretion occurs
- Areola: pigmented area surrounding the nipple
- Montgomery's glands: sebaceous gland located in the nipple and areola which secrete fluid to keep the areola and nipples moist and protected so that the tissue does not dry out
- The rest of the breast tissue consists of fatty and connective tissues.

Female genitalia

The structures of the normal external genitalia in a postpubertal woman are as follows:

- Vulva: the external visible parts of the female genitalia, bordered anteriorly by the symphysis pubis, laterally by the left and right thighs, and posteriorly by the buttocks
- Mons pubis: pad of fatty tissue overlying the symphysis pubis, covered by pubic hair
- Labia majora: two thick longitudinal folds of fatty tissue that form the lateral boundaries of the vulval (pudendal) cleft
- Labia minora: two folds of fatty tissue thinner than and lying parallel and medial to the labia majora
- Clitoris: small body of erectile tissue located at the superior junction of the labia majora
- Vestibule: the entrance to the vagina; contains the hymen, Skene's glands, and Bartholin's glands
- Fourchette: the posterior junction of the labia
- Perineum: area between the fourchette and the anus

Pelvic floor muscles

Levator ani, which is divided into three parts:

- Iliococcygeus muscle: supports the pelvic viscera and resist increases in intra-abdominal pressure
- Ischiococcygeus muscle: supports the pelvic viscera and resists increases in intra-abdominal pressure
- Pubococcygeus muscle: supports the pelvic viscera and resists increases in intra-abdominal pressure. This muscle is subdivided into three separate structures:
  - Pubovaginalis muscle: the most medial of the fibers of the pubococcygeus muscle; supports the anterior pelvic viscera
  - Puborectalis muscle: fibers that provide a sling for the rectum
  - Pubococcygeus muscle proper: controls urination and aids in childbirth

- 85 -

Major perineal muscles

The following are the perineal muscles:

- Bulbocavernosus muscle: surrounds the vagina and acts as a weak sphincter, closing the vagina and emptying the urethra. The bulbocavernosus also covers the vestibular bulbs, aggregations of erectile tissue that form a part of the clitoris.
- Ischiocavernosus muscle (ICM): helps maintain the erection of the clitoris

Note: The bulbocavernosus muscle and the ICM are the main muscles used during sexual intercourse. The contractions of these two muscles help in milking the semen from the penis into the vagina during penile withdrawal after ejaculation. In addition, steady contractions of these muscles occur with orgasm and may assist with ejaculation.

- Superficial and deep transverse perineal muscles: converge with the urethral sphincter and provide support for the perineum and the pelvic diaphragm
- External anal sphincter (EAS): barring pathology, the EAS is always in a state of contraction, keeping the anal canal and orifice closed.

Cervix

The cervix is the inferior portion of the uterus which joins at the proximal end of the vagina. The cervix consists of the following:

- Os: the opening in the center of the cervix which provides access into the uterine cavity and egress of the fetus during childbirth
- Squamocolumnar junction (SCJ): the border between the squamous epithelium of the body of the cervix (the ectocervix) and the columnar epithelium of the endocervix (the passageway between the cervical os and the uterine cavity)
- Transformation zone: the SCJ can change during the reproductive years. The area between the original site of the SCJ and its new site is called the transition zone (TZ). The TZ is important because dysplasia generally occurs in this area.

Vagina, fallopian tubes, and ovaries

The internal pelvic structures generally reach adult size and appearance by the time a woman reaches the age of sixteen:

- Vagina: muscular canal that connects the external genitalia with the cervix. Lined with stratified squamous epithelium. The wall of the vagina consists of rugae (folds) that allow the vagina to expand during sexual intercourse and childbirth. The pH is acidic because of the presence of lactobacilli.
- Fallopian tubes: tubes that transport the egg from the ovaries to the uterus via cilia that line the lumen of the tube. Each tube is approximately 10 cm long. The main body of the tube is the isthmus, the ampulla receives the egg at ovulation, and the ends of the tubes are fimbriated (fringed).
- Ovaries: egg-producing endocrine organs found at the ends of the fallopian tubes. The ovaries not only produce eggs but also produce estrogen and progesterone. Each ovary is approximately 3 x 2 x 1 cm in size.

- 86 -

Changes between puberty and adolescence

The hormonal sequence of events, physical changes, and psychosocial changes that occur between puberty and adolescence are as follows:

- Hormonal changes
  - The hypothalamic-pituitary-ovarian axis matures.
  - Gonadotropin-releasing hormone (GnRH) is released from the hypothalamus. GnRH causes the release of follicle-stimulating hormone (FSH) and luteinizing hormone (LH) from the anterior pituitary gland. FSH causes estrogen to be released from the ovaries. This results in the occurrence of secondary sexual characteristics and menstruation.
- Physical changes
  - Growth spurt takes place; the greatest velocity occurs just before the onset of menses.
  - Breast development (thelarche) begins with breast budding when the girl reaches approximately nine years of age; breasts are fully developed when she reaches approximately 17 years of age.
  - Growth of pubic and axillary hair (adrenarche) usually starts after breast development begins.
  - Menstruation starts when the girl reaches an average age of 12.5 years.
- Psychosocial changes
  - Development of struggle with independence and authority
  - Experimentation helps develop cognition.
  - Self-esteem develops.
  - Establishment of peer relationships

Tanner Staging system

The Tanner Staging system describes the physical development of the male and female on the basis of primary and secondary sex characteristics. The Tanner Stages based on pubic hair and breast development in the female are as follows:

- Pubic hair
  - Stage I: no pubic hair (prepubertal)
  - Stage II: small amount of downy-type hair with slight pigmentation on labia majora (10-11years)
  - Stage III: hair becomes curly and bristly, and lateral extension begins (12-14 years)
  - Stage IV: hair resembles adult hair but spares medial thighs (13-15 years)
  - Stage V: hair extends to medial thighs (16+ years)
- Breasts
  - Stage I: no glandular tissue; areola is not elevated from chest (prepubertal)
  - Stage II: breast bud forms under nipple, and areola begins to increase in diameter
  - Stage III: breast begins to elevate, extending beyond areola; however, areola is not elevated from breast
  - Stage IV: breast increases in size and elevation; areola forms mound projecting above breast tissue
  - Stage V: breast reaches adult size, areola returns to same level of breast

Menstrual cycle

The menstrual cycle and the phases that are involved in this cycle are described below:

- Ovarian cycle
  - Follicular phase:
    - ❖ Considered Day 1 of menstrual cycle
    - ❖ FSH/LH production increases, followed by
    - ❖ Drop in FSH with surge of LH about 12 hours before ovulation
  - Ovulation
    - ❖ Follicular capsule degraded by prostaglandins and proteolytic enzymes. Oocyte released. Cervical mucus thins
    - ❖ Sexual desire increases
  - Luteal phase
    - ❖ Ruptured follicle transformed into corpus luteum, which begins to secrete progesterone
    - ❖ Cervical mucus thickens
    - ❖ Corpus luteum deteriorates and progesterone declines if no pregnancy develops
    - ❖ Menses begins
- Uterine cycle
  - Proliferative change begins with estrogen secretion
    - ❖ Thickness of endometrium increases
  - Secretory phase begins with influence of progesterone
    - ❖ Endometrium continues to thicken
    - ❖ Vascularity increases
    - ❖ Uterine wall now prepared for implantation of zygote

Hormones

The origins and effects of the various hormones are listed below:

- Luteinizing hormone (LH): released from the pituitary in response to the production of GnRH by the hypothalamus. A surge of luteinizing hormone is responsible for ovulation in a dominant follicle and for follicular atresia in nondominant follicles.
- Prolactin: produced by the anterior pituitary gland. Prolactin is progressively released during pregnancy and results in the formation of milk.
- Gonadotropin-releasing hormone (GnRH): GnRH is released from the hypothalamus and stimulates the anterior pituitary gland to release FSH and LH.
- Adrenal hormones: released by the adrenal cortex
  - Cortisol: assists in the metabolism of fats, proteins, and carbohydrates
  - Aldosterone: regulates sodium (Na) and potassium (K) via the kidneys
  - Androstenedione: converts to estrone in fatty tissue
- Estrogen: produced by ovarian follicles, adrenal cortex, and corpus luteum; responsible for development of secondary sexual characteristics
- Estradiol: produced by ovarian follicles; the most important estrogen of reproductive age
- Estrone: the estrogen of menopause; results from the conversion of androstenedione, which is produced by the adrenal gland and ovarian stroma, to estrone at menopause

- Estriol: the estrogen of pregnancy; derived from the transformation of estrone and estradiol in the liver, uterus, placenta, and fetal adrenal glands
- Progesterone: produced by the ovarian corpus luteum; thickens the lining of the uterus and the cervical mucus
- Follicle-stimulating hormone (FSH): released from the pituitary gland in response to the production of GnRH by the hypothalamus; stimulates follicular growth in the ovary

Climacteric

The following are the physical changes to the breasts, skin, and bone integrity that occur during the climacteric:

- Breasts: as estrogen levels decrease, the fatty tissue in the breast is reabsorbed; this decreases the size of the breasts, giving them a flattened and pendulous appearance. The fibrous bands that support the breast become conspicuous.
- Skin: as the estrogen level decreases, the skin becomes thinner, less supple, and drier because the activity of the sebaceous glands and sweat glands decreases. The subcutaneous fatty tissue thins, which increases wrinkling and friability of the skin. Nonuniform hypopigmentation or hyperpigmentation can occur, as can thinning of scalp, pubic, and axillary hair.
- Bone integrity: with the decrease in estrogen, osteoporosis can develop. Bone loss accelerates as much as ten-fold, thereby increasing the risk of fractures.

The following are the physical changes to the reproductive organs and the urinary system that occur during the climacteric:

- Reproductive organs
  - Labia: the amount of fatty tissue decreases, as does tissue suppleness
  - Vagina: epithelial tissue thins, number of rugae decreases, and pH increases. Because of these changes, women may experience itching, painful intercourse (dyspareunia), and a white discharge (leukorrhea). The susceptibility to vaginitis may be increased.
  - Cervix: the size of the cervix and cervical os may decrease. The os may close (stenosis).
  - Uterus and ovaries: the uterus and ovaries may become smaller; the ovaries may become nonpalpable.
- Urinary system
  - Because of decreased muscle tone and atrophic changes in the urethral tissue, stress incontinence may develop.
  - Because of low estrogen levels, the ability to sense the need to void may decrease, resulting in stress urge incontinence.
  - Atrophic changes in the urethra may result in dysuria and frequency of urination.

Menopause

The following are the changes that occur to mood, cognition, libido, and quality of sleep during menopause:

- Mood changes: although most women do not experience psychological problems during menopause, a previous depression can resurface, perhaps because of the decreased sleep quality often associated with hot flashes. Hormonal changes can also result in anxiety, moodiness, and irritability.

- Cognition: forgetfulness and inability to concentrate are not uncommon, perhaps because of the decreased quality of sleep associated with nighttime hot flashes.
- Libido: because of changes in the structure of the vaginal and genital tissue during menopause, the woman perceives less sensation, which can lead to a change in the orgasm experience or to dyspareunia. Medication use and chronic illness may also affect libido. Conversely, increased privacy as the children leave home, no reason to fear pregnancy, and freedom from contractive use may increase sexual enjoyment.
- Sleep quality: Difficulty falling asleep or early wakening may occur, even if the woman is not experiencing hot flashes.

The following are the vasomotor and cardiovascular changes that may occur during menopause:

- Vasomotor symptoms: approximately 75% of women experience vasomotor symptoms, also known as "hot flashes." The cause of hot flashes is unknown, but their occurrence decreases as the woman ages. The symptoms of hot flashes are not just sensory; skin temperature actually increases during an episode. These episodes are extremely uncomfortable and are associated with profuse sweating and palpitations. Hot flashes can occur during sleep, waking the woman and resulting in insomnia, decreased sleep quality, and daytime fatigue. Loss of REM sleep can lead to cognitive dysfunction and anxiety disorders.
- Cardiovascular effects: increases in low density lipoprotein (LDL), very low density lipoprotein (VLDL), and triglyceride concentrations can lead to atherosclerosis. Clotting processes can be affected, with an increase in the activity of enzymes that dissolve fibrin, a protein essential for the clotting of blood. The production of procoagulation factors, also essential to the coagulation of blood, can also increase.

Perimenopausal and postmenopausal women

Screening

The following are the screening tests and other assessments that are necessary for perimenopausal and postmenopausal women:

- Pap smear every one to three years
- Annual rectal examination with fecal occult blood (FOB) test beginning when the woman reaches the age of 50
- Referral to gastroenterologist for colonoscopy when the woman reaches the age of 50. Gastroenterologist will determine when and how often follow-up colonoscopy should be performed.
- Annual mammogram beginning when the woman reaches the age of 40. Cholesterol, HDL, and LDL concentrations measured every 5 years, with follow-up laboratory tests depending on results
- Glucose and hemoglobin A1C (HA1C) every three years beginning when the woman reaches the age of 45, with follow-up depending on results
- Thyroid function tests every three to five years beginning when the woman reaches the age of 65. Screening should start when the woman is younger than 65 if there is a family history of thyroid disorders. A baseline hearing test should be done for any woman 65 years and older.
- Refer the woman to an ophthalmologist or optometrist when she reaches the age of 40 for evaluation for glaucoma and visual acuity. The ophthalmologist or optometrist will determine the frequency of follow-up.

<u>History and physical assessment</u>

The focus of a history and physical assessment as part of the overall health assessment of the perimenopausal or postmenopausal woman is described below:

- Health history
  - Focus on familial history of cancer, heart disease, depression, and osteoporosis.
  - Evaluate risk factors such as smoking, sexual behavior, alcohol, and drug use. Determine risk of sexually transmitted disease and HIV.
  - Menstrual history should include history of bleeding patterns and problems.
  - Evaluate nutrition and exercise patterns.
  - Psychosocial assessment should include questions about sexual satisfaction with partner, family or social support system, and history of sexual or domestic violence.
- Physical assessment
  - Vital signs, including blood pressure, height, and weight
  - Baseline body mass index (BMI) for comparison to future evaluations
  - Complete physical examination, including Pap smear and breast examination

Delayed puberty

While the onset of puberty varies, delayed puberty is no beginning of the development of secondary sexual characteristics (breast development, skeletal growth, increased pubic and axillary hair, increased body fat and changes in distribution, labial, uterine, and vaginal development) by age 13 in girls (and 14 in boys). Most girls begin breast development at about age 11 and experience menstruation by age 13. Some delay is related to a genetic predisposition, especially if a parent had delayed puberty. In some cases, delayed puberty can be caused by pituitary tumor that interferes with production of luteinizing hormone and follicle stimulating hormone, the hormones primarily responsible for development of secondary sexual characteristics. Some diseases are associated with retarded growth and delayed puberty, including sickle cell disease, cystic fibrosis, and chronic renal disease. PCOS may cause irregular periods, acne, and hirsutism. Turner syndrome, a genetic disease, may result in delayed puberty because of the lack of estrogen production.

Dysmenorrhea

Dysmenorrhea is defined as menstruation associated with lower abdominal cramping that may radiate to the back.

- Primary dysmenorrhea is not associated with any pelvic disease.
- Secondary dysmenorrhea is associated with any type of pelvic disease.

Signs and symptoms include cyclical pain beginning shortly after the onset of menses and lasting no longer than two days. Pain is located in the lower abdomen and occasionally radiates to the back. The differential diagnosis is long and may include imperforate hymen, endometriosis, cervical stenosis, uterine abnormalities, ovarian cysts, STDs, and UTIs. Assuming that secondary dysmenorrhea has been ruled out, management includes NSAIDs, oral contraceptives, exercise, or any combination of the three. If there is any reason to suspect a psychological etiology, the patient should be referred to a mental health specialist.

Premenstrual syndrome

Premenstrual syndrome (PMS) is defined as the cyclic occurrence of a group of physical and psychological symptoms that begin at ovulation and resolve after menses begins. The etiology of

PMS is unknown; because it may be a multifactorial and multiorgan disorder, many reasons for this condition have been suggested. Physical symptoms may include headache, breast tenderness, fluid retention, abdominal bloating, nausea, vomiting, food cravings, and lethargy. Psychological symptoms may include irritability, anxiety, depression, sleep alterations, anger, violent behavior, crying, and changes in libido. The symptoms may recur during the luteal phase. The findings of physical examination are usually normal. The differential diagnosis should include depression, anxiety, bipolar disorder, alcohol or drug abuse, diabetes, and thyroid disease. Laboratory tests should be ordered on the basis of the differential diagnosis. Management includes decreasing salt and caffeine intake, stopping alcohol intake, and increasing participation in exercise. Before antidepressants or anti-anxiety medications are prescribed, the patient should be seen by a mental health specialist.

Amenorrhea

Amenorrhea is defined as inappropriate absence of menses.

- Primary amenorrhea is defined as no history of previous menses; no menses by the age of 14, with the absence of development of secondary sexual characteristics; or no menses by the age of 16 regardless of secondary sexual characteristics.
- Secondary amenorrhea is the cessation of menses in a woman with a history of regular periods.

The differential diagnosis is extensive and includes vaginal agenesis, infection, genetic abnormalities, imperforate hymen, stress, medication effects, weight abnormalities, pregnancy, menopause, chronic illness, anorexia nervosa, and endocrine abnormalities. If a secondary cause for amenorrhea is suspected, that cause must be addressed first. If the diagnosis is primary amenorrhea, the patient should be referred to an endocrinologist.

DUB

Dysfunctional uterine bleeding (DUB) is defined as a variety of menstrual problems resulting from chronic anovulation. Risk factors include weight problems, chronic illness, excessive stress, and thyroid disease. The problem usually occurs during adolescence or during the climacteric. The signs and symptoms include any bleeding pattern that is outside the range of normal. The findings of physical examination are usually normal. The differential diagnosis includes pregnancy (either uterine or ectopic), cervical or uterine cancer, polycystic ovarian disease, liver disease, hematological disease, vaginitis, foreign body in the vagina (such as retained tampon), medication effects, drug abuse, and stress. Laboratory tests should include ßHCG test, Pap test, CBC, determination of FSH and LH levels, TFTs, STD tests, endometrial biopsy, cervical curettage to detect malignancy, and coagulation tests. Management includes use of oral contraceptive pills (OCPs), treatment of anemia if present, hysterectomy, dilation and curettage, and endometrial ablation.

Vulvovaginal candidiasis

Candidiasis is defined as inflammation of the vagina and vulva by yeast organisms, usually *Candida* species. Risk factors include diabetes, frequent intercourse, antibiotic use, and immunosuppressive disorders. Signs and symptoms may include itching, dysuria, edema, redness, dyspareunia, and a discharge that may be thin and watery or thick, resembling cottage cheese. Physical examination may reveal a discharge that adheres to the wall of the vagina and redness of the vaginal and vulval tissue. The differential diagnosis includes trichomoniasis, bacterial vaginosis, allergic reaction, and vulvar dermatitis. The diagnosis is made with a KOH wet prep, which will show mycelia, spores, and hyphae. The Pap smear may also detect fungal organisms. Management includes the use of antifungal vaginal creams or oral fluconazole (Diflucan). If the patient has persistent or recurrent candidiasis, she should be evaluated for diabetes or immunosuppressive disorders.

Candidiasis ("yeast infection"):

- Causative organism is *Candida* family of yeast, usually *Candida albicans*
- *C. albicans* is a normal flora, but the fungus proliferates and can cause vaginal symptoms when conditions that keep the number of organisms in check are affected.
- Risk factors
  - Diabetes
  - Stress
  - Fatigue
  - Antibiotic use
  - General illness
  - HIV infection
- Signs and symptoms
  - Vaginal itching
  - Vaginal soreness
  - Red, swollen vulva
  - Dyspareunia
  - Dysuria
  - Thick, cottage cheese–like discharge
- Diagnosis - Wet prep with KOH will show typical fungal hyphae
- Treatment
  - Miconazole (Monistat) vaginal suppository, one at bedtime for one to three days (Pregnancy Category C)
  - Terconazole (Terazol) vaginal suppository, one at bedtime for three consecutive nights (Pregnancy Category C)

Bacterial vaginosis

Bacterial vaginosis (BV) is defined as an alteration of the normal vaginal flora. BV may be caused by a host of different organisms, including *Gardnerella vaginalis*, *Mycoplasma hominis*, and *Haemophilus* species. Risk factors include STDs, multiple sex partners, and the use of IUDs. Signs and symptoms of BV include occasional itching and a vaginal discharge that may be grayish, yellowish, or whitish, has a rancid odor, and may coat the vulva. The differential diagnosis includes yeast infection or Trichomoniasis infection. Diagnostic tests include a wet mount of the vaginal secretions to determine the presence of clue cells (epithelial cells with the borders ill-defined because of the presence of bacteria) and the detection of a fishy odor ("whiff test") after 10% KOH solution is added to a slide of the discharge. Management includes metronidazole (Flagyl) three times daily for seven days, metronidazole vaginal cream at bedtime for five days, or clindamycin twice daily for seven days.

Bacterial vaginosis is acquired when the normal balance of vaginal bacteria is disrupted.

- Risk factors
  - Multiple sex partners

- o Douching
- o Use of an IUD
- Complications
  - o Increased risk of acquiring HIV infection if patient has sex with a patient who has HIV
  - o Increased chance of passing on HIV infection if patient has HIV infection
  - o Increased risk of pelvic inflammatory disease (PID)
  - o Increased risk of complications if pregnant
  - o Increased susceptibility to other STDs
  - o Increased risk of delivering a baby with low birth weight
- Signs and symptoms
  - o Vaginal itching or burning
  - o Thin gray or white vaginal discharge
  - o Foul, fishy odor
- Diagnosis
  - o Clue cells found on wet prep
  - o Vaginal fluid pH 4.5 or higher
  - o Vaginal discharge
- Treatment
  - o Metronidazole (Flagyl) one dose of 2.0 gm (Pregnancy Category B), OR
  - o Clindamycin (Cleocin) vaginal cream, one applicator-full at bedtime for seven days (Pregnancy Category B)

Diagnosis of STDs

The screening tests used to diagnose *Chlamydia trachomatis, Neisseria gonorrhea*, and syphilis are as follows:

- Chlamydia trachomatis
  - o Culture of tissue from cervix, vagina, rectum, and pharynx
  - o DNA culture
- Neisseria gonorrhea
  - o DNA culture. Culture of tissue from cervix, vagina, vulva, rectum, and pharynx. Enzyme-linked immunosorbent assay (ELISA)
- Treponema pallidum (syphilis)
  - o Dark-field microscopy (DFM) and direct fluorescent antibody (DFA) tests of exudate from lesion
  - o Serological tests (nontreponemal)
    - ❖ Venereal Disease Research Laboratory (VDRL) test
    - ❖ Rapid plasma reagin (RPR) test
    - ❖ Note: Any positive nontreponemal test result must be verified by a treponemal test. Also, after the patient has been treated, nontreponemal tests become nonreactive over time, and some false-positives may occur if the patient has collagen vascular disease or mononucleosis.
  - o Serological tests (treponemal)
    - ❖ Fluorescent treponemal antibody absorption test (FTA-ABS)

❦ Treponema pallidum immobilization test (TPI)

❦ Note: Unlike nontreponemal test results, treponemal test results remain positive after the patient has been treated.

The screening tests used to test for *Herpes simplex* virus (HSV) infection, human papillomavirus (HPV) infection, hepatitis B virus (HBV) infection, and human immunodeficiency virus (HIV) infection are as follows:

- HSV infection
  - A tissue culture of the lesion is the gold standard; however, most clinicians base the diagnosis of *Herpes* on clinical presentation.
    - ❖ Prodrome of itching or burning in area
    - ❖ Formation of fluid-filled vesicles on a red base
    - ❖ Rupture of vesicles forms a painful ulcerated lesion.
- HPV infection (genital warts)
  - Causative organism is *Condyloma acuminata.*
  - Diagnosis is based on clinical examination.
  - A punch biopsy can be performed to confirm the diagnosis but is rarely needed.
- HBV infection
  - Hepatitis B surface antigen (HBsAg) is seen in a patient with an active infection and in carriers of the disease.
  - Hepatitis B surface antibody (HBsAb) is seen as the infection resolves and confers immunity to HBV.
  - Hepatitis B core antibody (HBcAb) indicates chronic hepatitis.
- Human immunodeficiency virus (HIV) infection
  - ELISA test nonspecific
  - If ELISA is positive, Western blot testing must be performed to confirm infection.

Trichomoniasis

Trichomoniasis is a vaginal infection caused by the parasite *Trichomonas*. Trichomoniasis is considered a sexually transmitted disease; although transmission by fomites is theoretically possible, it is unlikely. Risk factors include multiple sex partners, the presence of another STD, and failure to use condoms. Signs and symptoms of trichomoniasis include a copious, greenish or yellowish vaginal discharge, associated with itching and edema. Urinary frequency, postcoital bleeding, and dysuria may occur. Physical examination may reveal a swollen, red, painful vulva; red stippling ("strawberry spots") on the vagina and cervix; vaginal discharge; or a friable cervix. The infection can spread to the Bartholin's glands, the endocervix, and the periurethral glands. The differential diagnosis includes bacterial vaginosis, yeast infection, and trauma from insertion of a foreign body. Diagnostic tests include a saline wet mount to visualize the parasite. The parasite may also be detected by a Pap test. Management involves metronidazole twice a daily for seven days.

Trichomoniasis:

- Infectious organism is the parasite Trichomonas vaginalis
- Acquired during sexual intercourse with an infected partner
- Complications
  - Increased susceptibility to HIV infection
  - Increased risk of passing on HIV if patient has HIV infection

- o   Possible increased susceptibility to other STDs
- o   Premature rupture of the membranes
- o   Preterm delivery, Low birth weight
- Signs and symptoms
  - o   Frothy, yellow-green vaginal discharge
  - o   Foul odor
  - o   Vaginal itching
  - o   Dysuria
  - o   Dyspareunia
- Diagnosis
  - o   Flagellated, oval-shaped organisms seen under a light microscope are pathognomonic of "Trich" infection.
- Treatment
  - o   Metronidazole (Flagyl) one dose of 2.0 gm (Pregnancy Category B), OR
  - o   Metronidazole (Flagyl) 500 mg twice daily for seven days (Pregnancy Category B)

Chlamydia and gonorrhea

Chlamydia and gonorrhea are sexually transmitted diseases; chlamydia is caused by the *Chlamydia trachomatis* organism, and gonorrhea is caused by the *Neisseria gonorrhea* organism. Chlamydia is the most common STD in the United States. Four million cases of chlamydia and as many as 2 million cases of gonorrhea are reported annually. Risk factors for both diseases include sexually activity by women who unmarried and younger than 25 years, multiple sex partners, a history of STDs, and the use of birth control pills. The signs and symptoms of chlamydia may include postcoital bleeding, dysuria, vaginal discharge, and abdominal pain. Physical examination may show vaginal discharge, a friable cervix, and lower abdominal tenderness. Diagnostic tests used to determine the presence of chlamydia and gonorrhea include cell cultures (expensive), enzyme immunoassay (EIA), polymerase chain reaction (PCR), and the nucleic acid amplification test (NAAT). NAAT uses PCR and is the easiest to use, requiring only a urine specimen. Management includes azithromycin, one 2.0-gm dose. The patient should also be treated for gonorrhea and tested for syphilis and HIV.

- Risk factors
  - o   Prostitution
  - o   Sexual abuse
  - o   Poverty
  - o   Adolescence
  - o   Drug abuse
  - o   Associated STD
  - o   Multiple partners
- Signs and symptoms
  - o   May have symptoms of vaginal discharge or dysuria
  - o   Dyspareunia
  - o   Many cases are asymptomatic.

Pelvic inflammatory disease results when organism migrates to uterus or tubes, with associated fever, abdominal pain, nausea, and vomiting. It is often associated with chlamydia.

- Diagnosis
  - Gram stain, DNA probe, Gonorrhea culture
  - Always treat for concomitant chlamydia.
- Treatment
  - Ceftriaxone sodium (Rocephin), one dose of 250 mg IM (Pregnancy Category B) for the Neisseria gonorrhoeae organism
  - Azithromycin (Zithromax), one dose of 2.0 gm (Pregnancy Category B) for the Chlamydia trachomatis organism
  - If patient is allergic to either of these medications, contact local Public Health Department for treatment recommendations for local area.
  - Patient's sexual partner(s) should also be treated to prevent reinfection and spread of the disease.

Syphilis

Syphilis is a sexually transmitted disease caused by the organism *Treponema pallidum.* Syphilis has four stages:

- Primary: involves the formation of a chancre at the site of entry of the organism; the chancre is painless and may not be noticed.
- Secondary: involves systemic spread with many types of skin manifestations (generally on soles and palms), along with flu-like symptoms.
- Latent: at this stage, the disease is asymptomatic.
- Tertiary stage: involves affliction of any organ system, such as neurological (meningitis, paralysis, insanity) or cardiovascular (aortitis, aneurysm).

Diagnosis includes serological testing (VDRL, RPR) or dark-field microscopy of the fluid from a syphilitic lesion; these tests will reveal the organisms. Management includes the use of azithromycin, ciprofloxin, erythromycin, or ceftriaxone.

Primary syphilis:

- Incubation period approximately 6 weeks
- Genital lesion easy to miss; usually appears as a painless ulcer (the chancre), Ulcer will heal after several weeks without treatment.
- Patient may have nontender inguinal lymphadenopathy.

Secondary syphilis

- Characterized by diverse skin lesions (especially on palms and soles) that may be transient or may last for several months
- Generalized symptoms may appear flu-like
- Scattered alopecia, appearing "moth-eaten"
- Possible condylomata lata, which are highly infectious

Tertiary (latent) syphilis

- May be asymptomatic, although still infectious
- Neurosyphilis: deterioration of motor function, dementia, emotional lability, tremors. Cardiovascular syphilis: thoracic aneurysms, valvular insufficiency

Diagnosis:

- VDRL or RPR should be included in prenatal laboratory workup.
- If results of either test are positive, confirm with FTA-ABS.

Treatment:

- Benzathine penicillin G, 2.4 million units IM, with second dose in one week. If patient is allergic to penicillin, contact local Public Health Department for treatment recommendations for local area.

HSV

Herpes simplex (HSV) is a recurrent, incurable viral infection of the skin. HSV-1 usually is found in the orolabial region, whereas HSV-2 is found in the genital area; however, sexual practices are blurring this distinction. Approximately 45 million Americans are affected, and approximately 1 million new cases are diagnosed annually. The first outbreak may include the following signs and symptoms: fever, lymphadenopathy, headache, and other "flu-like" symptoms before the outbreak of vesicles on a raised red base at the site of entry of the virus. Subsequent breakouts generally lack the constitutional symptoms; a prodrome of itching or tingling may precede the outbreak of the herpetic lesion. The main concern associated with the presence of the herpes lesion during delivery is infection of the infant, which could be fatal. Management includes oral antiviral agents such as acyclovir, famciclovir, and valacyclovir. If a woman in labor has a herpetic lesion that may come into contact with the baby, a cesarean section is indicated.

Herpes simplex virus (HSV):

- Signs and symptoms
  - Prodrome of itching, burning, or fullness at site of inoculation
  - Small vesicles on a raised, red base
  - Flu-like symptoms
  - Vesicles break, leaving a shallow, painful ulcer.
  - Associated inguinal lymphadenopathy
  - Ulcer heals in two to four weeks.
  - Lesion may recur, usually at same site, if patient is under stress, is exposed to bright sunlight, or is fatigued.
- Diagnosis
  - Tzanck test is the gold standard but is usually unnecessary. Diagnosis can be made on basis of history and presentation of the herpetic lesion.
  - Blood tests cannot indicate when infection was acquired.
- Treatment
  - Acyclovir (Pregnancy Category B)
  - Valacyclovir (Pregnancy Category B)
  - Famciclovir (Pregnancy Category B)

Condyloma acuminata

Condyloma acuminata is (venereal warts) a sexually transmitted viral disease that can affect the cervix, vagina, vulva, perineum, and anus. The disease is caused by the human papillomavirus (HPV), which is associated with abnormal cytologic findings in 80% to 90% of cases. Risk factors include smoking, multiple sex partners, early first intercourse, history of an STD, low socioeconomic status, and diseases that suppress the immune system. Signs and symptoms include wart-like lesions that can be flat, elevated, pedunculated, or cauliflower-like in appearance. The differential diagnosis includes carcinoma, skin tags, molluscum contagiosum, and other skin disorders. Management includes colposcopy, cryotherapy, and topical agents. If lesion is suspicious, a biopsy is indicated to determine malignant potential.

UTI

Urinary tract infection (UTI) is defined as an infection in any part of the urinary system, such as cystitis (bladder infection), urethritis (infection of the urethra) or pyelonephritis (kidney infection). *E. coli* is the most common causative organism. Risk factors include renal failure, diabetes, pregnancy, renal calculi, poor hygiene, infrequent voiding, inadequate fluid intake, frequent intercourse, sickle cell disease, catheterization, and douching. Signs and symptoms can be mild to severe and may include dysuria, frequency, urgency, suprapubic discomfort, hematuria, costovertebral angle tenderness, fever, nausea, and vomiting. The differential diagnosis includes vaginitis, STD, renal calculi, and neoplasm. Diagnosis involves microscopy of urine, which will show white blood cells and bacteria. Urine C&S should also be ordered. Management includes the use of antibiotics for three to five days. The choice of antibiotic should be based on the locally predominant pathogens. The patient should be encouraged to increase water intake and to minimize the intake of caffeine (a diuretic).

- Cystitis (bladder infection)
  - Suprapubic discomfort
  - Dysuria
  - Frequency
  - Urgency
- Pyelonephritis (infection has spread to the kidneys)
  - Fever/chills
  - Lower unilateral or bilateral back pain
  - Nausea/vomiting
  - Dysuria
  - General malaise
- Diagnosis
  - Physical examination
    - ❖ Unilateral or bilateral CVA tenderness upon percussion of area
    - ❖ Tender suprapubic area or lower abdomen
  - Dipstick urine test results
    - ❖ Positive for leukocytes
    - ❖ Positive for nitrite
    - ❖ Positive for protein
- Management of simple cystitis
  - Send urine for culture and sensitivity (C&S) testing

- o Pending results of C&S - Nitrofurantoin (Macrobid) 100 mg every 12 hours for 7 days (Pregnancy Category B) OR Cephalexin (Keflex) 500 mg twice daily for 7 to 10 days (Pregnancy Category B) AND
- o Phenazopyridine HCL (Pyridium) 200 mg three times daily for 5 days (Pyridium is a urinary tract anesthetic.)
- o Patient should increase fluid intake
- o Some women claim improvement with drinking cranberry juice.
- o Check patient again in ten days.
- o If recurrent UTIs are a problem, consider suppressive therapy.

PID

Pelvic inflammatory disease (PID) includes a spectrum of inflammatory disorders of the upper reproductive tract. The most common organisms associated with PID are *Chlamydia trachomatis, Neisseria gonorrhea,* and occasionally *E. coli, G. vaginalis,* and *H. influenzae.* One million cases are diagnosed annually, with 200,000 hospitalizations. Twenty-five percent of cases lead to infertility, ectopic pregnancy, and chronic pelvic pain. Risk factors include sexually activity by women younger 20 years, multiple sexual partners, history of previous PID, vaginal douching, and smoking. Signs and symptoms can include mild to severe abdominal pain, vaginal discharge, fever, dysuria, dyspareunia, nausea, and vomiting.

Physical examination may reveal lower abdominal tenderness, adnexal mass, high fever, and vaginal discharge. The differential diagnosis includes ectopic pregnancy, appendicitis, ruptured ovarian cyst, endometriosis, adnexal mass torsion, and renal calculi. Testing may include checking for chlamydia or gonorrheal infection, ultrasonography of abdomen, pelvis, or both, and laparoscopy. Management includes ofloxacin and metronidazole for 14 days. Hospitalization should be considered if the patient is pregnant, if pelvic abscess or ectopic pregnancy is suspected, if the patient is infected with HIV, or if the patient is an adolescent.

Endometriosis

Endometriosis is the presence of endometrial tissue outside the uterus. The etiology of endometriosis is unclear but may include retrograde menses, immunological factors, genetic predisposition, and hormonal factors. It occurs in women of all races and ages; however, the typical patient is 20 to 30 years old, Caucasian, and nulliparous. Although most extrauterine tissue is found in the pelvis, such tissue can also be found anywhere in the body, including the lungs, nose, and spinal column. The signs and symptoms vary but may include dysmenorrhea, infertility, premenstrual spotting, pelvic pain, dyspareunia, back pain, and dysuria. Symptoms usually occur at or just before menses. The physical examination may show a fixed uterus, tender adnexal masses, nodular uterosacral ligaments, and visible lesions on laparoscopy. The differential diagnosis includes acute or chronic PID, ectopic pregnancy, and ovarian neoplasm. Management includes analgesics, oral contraceptives, laser surgery, and hysterectomy.

Infertility

Infertility is defined as failure to conceive after one year of unprotected sexual intercourse. Female factors may include ovulatory dysfunction, polycystic ovaries, ovarian failure, fibroids, neoplasm, congenital abnormalities, salpingitis, endometriosis, cervicitis, DES exposure in utero, thyroid disease, infrequent coitus, and smoking cigarettes or marijuana. The incidence of infertility increases as the woman and her oocytes age. Male factors may include oligospermia, presence of sperm antibodies, environmental exposure to toxins, use of marijuana, cocaine use, DES exposure, infrequent coitus, and varicocele. Diagnostic tests may include hysterosalpingogram and hysteroscopy. Huhner's test for postcoital evaluation of the sperm count and quality may be considered. Management is determined by the diagnosis. Hormone therapy or surgery may be considered for the woman; surgery may be considered for the man. In vitro fertilization (IVF) may be an option and, if so, should be discussed with the couple.

2001 Bethesda System for reporting cervical cytology

The 2001 Bethesda System for reporting cervical cytology (Pap test) is as follows:

- Specimen adequacy
  - Satisfactory: determined by presence of endocervical and transformation zone components
  - Unsatisfactory: specimen obscured by blood or inadequate number of squamous cells
- Interpretation
  - Negative for malignancy, No epithelial cell abnormality
  - Presence of organisms such as Trichomonas, fungus, BV, HSV, Reactive cells consistent with inflammation
  - Epithelial cell abnormality - Squamous cell abnormalities: Atypical squamous cells of undetermined significance (ASCUS), Low-grade squamous intraepithelial lesion (LSIL) such as HPV, High-grade squamous intraepithelial lesion (HSIL) such as carcinoma in situ
  - Squamous cell carcinoma
  - Glandular cell abnormalities - Atypical glandular cells (AGC) specified as endocervical or endometrial, Atypical glandular cells favoring neoplasia
- Management of a woman whose Pap test has returned abnormal results is determined by those results. If organisms are present, the appropriate medication should be prescribed. Any structural abnormality should be referred for gynecological evaluation.

Uterine fibroids

Uterine fibroids, the most common benign gynecologic pelvic neoplasm, are nodular tumors ranging in size from microscopic to large masses. They affect approximately 20% of women and are more common among African Americans than among Caucasians. Asymptomatic masses may occur in 40% to 50% of women aged 40 or older. Fibroids are classified according to their location:

- Submucosal fibroids protrude into the uterine cavity.
- Subserosal fibroids bulge through the uterine wall.
- Intraligamentous fibroids are within the broad ligament.
- Interstitial or intramural fibroids stay within the uterine wall as they grow.
- Pedunculated fibroids are found on a thin pedicle attached to the uterus.

Signs and symptoms of uterine fibroids may include excessive bleeding during menses, chronic pelvic pain, dyspareunia, and constipation or intestinal obstruction if the tumors are large.

Physical examination may reveal abdominal enlargement, an enlarged or displaced uterus, or a pedunculated tumor protruding from the cervix. The tumors are usually painless upon palpation. The differential diagnosis includes benign or malignant ovarian or uterine mass, pregnancy, endometriosis, and benign or malignant colon or rectal tumor. Diagnostic tests include Pap test, ßHCG test, CBC to rule out anemia, fecal occult blood test to rule out colorectal involvement, abdominal or pelvic ultrasound or both, CT or MRI, endometrial biopsy, D&C, or hysteroscopy. Management includes only monitoring if lesions are asymptomatic. It is imperative that the patient undergo periodic Pap tests and bimanual examinations to ensure that the tumors are not growing or undergoing any abnormal changes. Hormonal pharmacotherapy may decrease the size of the masses. Anemia needs to be treated if present. Surgery, such as hysterectomy, may be considered if the patient is experiencing abnormal bleeding, if the fibroids are growing rapidly, or if the mass or masses begin to encroach on other organs.

Adenomyosis

Adenomyosis occurs when endometrial tissue lining the uterus invades the myometrium, resulting in areas of endometrial tissue within the uterine wall. Adenomyosis is a secondary cause of dysmenorrhea and may be associated with endometriosis but is a separate condition. Typical indications include a tender, enlarged, and soft- or "boggy"-feeling uterus and dysmenorrhea. Women may experience heavy menstrual flow with clots, severe painful cramping during menses, bleeding between periods, and painful intercourse. Because the uterus may become very enlarged (two to three times the normal size), abdominal distention and discomfort may occur. Risk factors include history of Cesarean section (C-section), childbirth, or surgical removal of fibroids. Diagnosis is based on physical exam, ultrasound, and/or MRI. Treatment includes NSAIDs to control pain, estrogen–progestin oral contraceptives or progestin-only oral contraceptives or devices may control cycles to reduce pain. The only definitive treatment is hysterectomy, which may be an option if dysmenorrhea is severe and uncontrolled by more conservative measures.

Adnexal masses

Follicular cyst

Follicular cysts occur when levels of luteinizing hormone are insufficient to produce rupture of the ovarian follicle and ovulation. The cysts fill with fluid (estrogen-rich) and grow. Follicular cysts usually reabsorb within two to three months, but in some cases they may continue to grow and present as an asymptomatic adnexal mass, sometimes becoming large enough (> 5 cm) to result in mild to moderate pain in the right or left lower abdomen and changes in the menstrual cycle (irregular bleeding) because of overstimulation of the endometrium from subsequent failed ovulation and/or large amounts of estradiol produced by the cyst. In some cases, a ruptured follicular cyst may cause acute pain because follicular fluid is released into the peritoneum. Ultrasound is usually recommended for cysts > 5 cm, although smaller cysts may simply be reassessed manually in six weeks. A combined estrogen-progestin oral contraceptive may prevent development of further cysts.

Corpus luteum cyst

Once the ovum is released from a follicle following increased levels of lutein hormone, the follicle is called a corpus luteum, which produces increased levels of hormones (estrogen/progesterone). If the corpus luteum seals over and begins to enlarge to > 3 cm, it becomes a corpus luteum cyst. There are two types:

- Slightly enlarged cyst continues to produce progesterone, delaying menstruation by up to two weeks or longer. Persistent corpus luteum cysts are characterized by (i) delayed menstruation, (iii) dull pain in the lower quadrant, and (ii) adnexal enlargement. A pregnancy test should be done to rule out ectopic pregnancy. Cyclic oral contraceptives may relieve persistent corpus luteum cysts.

- Cyst with spontaneous internal hemorrhage rapidly enlarges during the luteal phase and may rupture, resulting in acute pain. Typically, women are not taking oral contraceptives and have normal periods. If symptoms of hemoperitoneum or hypovolemia occur, surgical resection may be needed to control bleeding, but most resolve without treatment other than analgesia.

Benign ovarian neoplasms

About a fourth of adnexal masses result from benign ovarian neoplasms. In women of reproductive age, 90% of these ovarian neoplasms are benign, while 75% are malignant in postmenopausal women. There are three primary types of benign tumors: epithelial cell, germ cell, and stromal cell:

- Epithelial cell: Includes the serous cystadenoma (most common), which may occur in any age group, especially ages 40 to 50. About 70% are benign, but because of the risk of malignancy, an ovarian cystectomy (for younger women) or oophorectomy is performed. In postmenopausal women, hysterectomy and bilateral oophorectomy may be done to reduce risk of recurrence or malignancy.
- Germ cell (cystic teratoma or dermoid): Germ cell tumors may contain differentiated tissues, such as hair, teeth, glandular tissue, or bone. The average age of occurrence is 30. The tumor is often asymptomatic except for an adnexal mass. Although malignancy is < 1%, the tumor is surgically removed because of high rates of ovarian torsion and rupture, which may cause peritonitis. About 10% to 20% are bilateral.

Benign ovarian neoplasms include stromal cell neoplasms in addition to epithelial cell and germ cell neoplasms. Most of these tumors develop from gonadal tissue, so they produce hormones. They may occur at any age and have the potential to become malignant, so they are surgically excised. The three primary types of stroma cell neoplasms include:

- Granulosa theca cell: Produce estrogenic components, resulting in increased feminization (and precocious puberty in children). Reproductive age women have heavy menstrual flow, and postmenopausal patients may experience vaginal bleeding. Occurrence is usually at 50 to 55 years.
- Sertoli–Leydig cell: Produce androgenic components, resulting in virilization, including hirsutism, and < 5% become malignant. Occurrence is usually in young adulthood (average age 25).
- Ovarian fibroma: Derive from collagen production of spindle cells and are most common during middle age, comprising 4% of ovarian tumors. This tumor does not produce hormones and is usually small and solid and may be associated with ascites and right pleural effusion (Meigs syndrome).

Cervical polyps

Cervical polyps are usually benign pedunculated growths on the surface of the cervix. Polyps are the most common benign lesions of the cervix. The cause may be inflammation, pregnancy, or trauma. These lesions are most common among perimenopausal and multigravida women aged 30 to 50 years. Signs and symptoms may include a white or clear vaginal discharge and abnormal vaginal bleeding, especially after intercourse. The physical examination will show single or multiple painless, friable, pedunculated lesions on the cervix ranging in size from a few millimeters to 2to 3 cm. The differential diagnosis includes carcinoma, sarcoma, retained products of conception, and prolapsed myoma. Diagnostic tests include a Pap smear and biopsy of the lesions. Colposcopy is usually indicated. Management includes excision of the lesions, although they frequently recur.

Endometrial polyps

Endometrial polyps are most common during the perimenopausal or postmenopausal period (40 to 50) and result from focal hyperplasia. They may be associated with other types of endometrial hyperplasia or carcinoma, although only about 5% slow malignant changes, more often in postmenopausal women than women of reproductive age. Polyps may vary in size (1 to 2 mm to 5 cm) and number and usually are not associated with pain unless they become large and protrude through the cervix, resulting in cervical dilation that may cause dull midline pain. The most common symptom is vaginal bleeding. Premenopausal women may experience irregular periods with heavy bleeding and/or bleeding between periods as well as infertility. Hypertension, obesity, and use of tamoxifen increase risks. Treatment includes watching and waiting, curettage, surgical excision, and hysterectomy. Medications (progestins and gonadotropin-releasing hormone agonists) may shrink polyps, but they grow again when the medication is stopped.

DES

Diethylstilbestrol (DES) is an estrogen that was prescribed to approximately 2 million women between 1942 and 1971 to prevent miscarriages. It was found that daughters of women who took DES have a higher incidence of vaginal cancer, cervical cancer, or both. Sons of women who took DES have a 25% chance of undescended testicles. Mechanism of action: The vagina of the fetus is lined with columnar epithelium. As the fetus matures, this columnar epithelium is replaced with squamous epithelium. DES exposure during this transformation prevents full development of the squamous epithelium. As many as 25% of women exposed to DES in utero experience structural changes in the reproductive system, such as transverse vaginal septum, cervical collar, or a uterine constricting band. All such problems are dose and time related: if DES was administered after the 18th week of gestation, the risk of these abnormalities is significantly higher. Patients with a vaginal lining of columnar epithelium instead of squamous epithelium are especially susceptible to human papillomavirus infection.

Signs and symptoms are few but may include dyspareunia, postcoital bleeding, and infertility problems. Physical findings may include areas of vaginal adenosis (columnar epithelium), vaginal or cervical nodularity, visible cervical abnormalities, and uterine abnormalities such as a T-shaped uterus or a bicornate uterus. Diagnostic tests include Pap smear, colposcopy with biopsy, and hysterosalpingogram or uterine ultrasonography to determine whether any uterine abnormalities are present. Management of DES-induced abnormalities includes regular Pap tests; regular bimanual examination of the vagina, cervix, and uterus to determine whether masses are present; and referral to a gynecologist.

Endometrial carcinoma

Endometrial carcinoma is defined as malignant transformation of the tissue of the uterus. Endometrial carcinoma is the most common type of gynecologic malignancy; 300,000 cases are diagnosed annually, and the condition causes 6,000 deaths each year. Risk factors include diabetes, obesity, hypertension, positive family history, early menarche, late menopause, unopposed estrogen therapy, and estrogen-secreting tumors. The signs and symptoms include painless vaginal bleeding, a watery vaginal discharge followed by a bloody discharge, and occasional abdominal pain. The physical examination may reveal blood in the vagina, pelvic mass, ascites, anemia, or an enlarged uterus. The differential diagnosis includes vaginitis, polyps, DUB, fibroids, and neoplasms. Diagnostic tests may include abdominal or pelvic ultrasound, Pap test, and diagnostic D&C. Management involves referral to a gynecological oncologist.

Cervical carcinoma

Cervical cancer is defined as the invasion of the basement membrane of the cervix by malignant cells. Approximately 14,500 new cases of cervical cancer are diagnosed each year, and approximately 4,500 women die of this disease annually. The highest incidence of death occurs among Hispanics, then among African Americans, and then among whites. Risk factors include smoking, human papilloma virus (HPV) infection, first sexual intercourse earlier than at the age of 18 years, multiple sex partners, low socioeconomic status, DES exposure, and multiparity. Signs and symptoms can include postcoital bleeding, irregular bleeding, a bloody, malodorous discharge, and pelvic pain. The disease may also be asymptomatic. The physical examination findings can range from a normal-appearing cervix to ulcerated, necrotic, or bulky lesions. The differential diagnosis includes metastasis, cervicitis, STD, polyps, and condyloma. Tests that should be ordered include Pap smear, biopsy of lesions, colposcopy, and CT, MRI, or both. Management involves referring the patient to a gynecological oncologist.

Vaginal carcinoma

Vaginal carcinoma is defined as invasion of the vaginal basement membrane by malignant cells. Signs and symptoms may include unusual vaginal bleeding, bloody discharge, itching, palpable mass, unexplained lesions, and urinary problems (if the bladder is involved). Physical examination may reveal white, raised, friable, granular, or cauliflower-like lesions. Tissue ulceration may also be present. The upper third of the vagina is the most common location of vaginal carcinoma. Melanoma should be suspected if the lesion is darkly pigmented. The differential diagnosis includes vaginitis, metastasis from a primary tumor in another organ system, endometriosis, and vaginal trauma due to insertion of a foreign body. Diagnostic tests include Pap test, colposcopy, evaluation of the gastrointestinal and urinary systems, and CT or MRI if metastasis is suspected. Management involves referral to a gynecologic oncologist, and possible gastroenterology and urology evaluation if metastasis is suspected.

Ovarian carcinoma

Ovarian carcinoma is defined as malignant transformation of the ovarian tissue. Risk factors include family history, low parity, early menarche, late menopause, high socioeconomic class, high fat consumption, and a history of breast, colon or endometrial cancer. Signs and symptoms are the following:

- Early stage: may be asymptomatic, or may cause abdominal discomfort or a feeling of pelvic fullness.
- Late stage: symptoms may include increasing abdominal girth, abdominal pain, abnormal vaginal bleeding, and gastrointestinal symptoms such as nausea or loss of appetite.

Physical examination may reveal a fixed, nontender, unilateral or bilateral adnexal mass, ascites, and general ill health, including unexplained weight loss. The differential diagnosis includes endometriosis, benign tumors, ovarian cyst, ovarian torsion, pelvic kidney, and fibroids. Diagnostic tests include abdominal and pelvic ultrasound and MRI, CT, or both. Definitive diagnosis requires laparotomy. Management requires referral to a gynecologic oncologist.

BSE

The following is the technique of the breast self examination (BSE), including its limitations:

- Inspection – observe for asymmetry, dimpling, or any other abnormalities
    - Stand in front of a mirror
    - Raise arms over head
    - Place hands on hips
    - Bend forward
- Palpation – checking for masses, lumps or anything unusual. One of several techniques can be used:
    - In shower or bath, wet and soap breasts, raise arm and check breast with opposite hand. Slipperiness of soap will increase chance of finding mass.
    - Lie in bed with pillow under shoulder, raise arm, and inspect breast with opposite hand.
        - ❖ Using pads of fingers, press and gently massage breast tissue against ribs
        - ❖ Imperative that entire breast is examined: medially to laterally from sternum to axilla and superiorly to inferiorly from clavicle to bottom of ribs
        - ❖ Several patterns of examination are acceptable:
            - Circular pattern
            - Grid pattern
            - Most important thing is that all breast tissue is inspected.

Breast carcinoma

Breast carcinoma is the most common female malignancy, and its incidence is increasing in the United States. Risk factors include the breast cancer genes BRCA 1 and BRCA 2, advancing age, family history of breast cancer, history of breast cancer, perimenopause, history of endometrial or colon cancer, menopause after the age of 55, nulliparity, obesity, radiation exposure, and heavy alcohol use. Signs and symptoms may include breast mass, nipple discharge of any type, changes in breast skin (dimpling, retraction, scaling, redness), and lymphadenopathy (axillary, supraclavicular, or infraclavicular). The differential diagnosis includes fibroadenoma, fibrocystic breast changes, trauma, mastitis, galactorrhea, medication side effects, pregnancy, shingles (herpes zoster), and chronic breast stimulation. Diagnostic tests may include ßHCG test, mammography, ultrasonography to determine whether mass is cystic or solid, CT/MRI to rule out metastasis, and biopsy. The definitive diagnosis is made by results of histological testing of a specimen obtained by fine-needle aspiration (FNA), open biopsy, or needle biopsy. Management is referral to an oncologist for staging and treatment.

Fibroadenoma

Fibroadenoma is a benign breast lesion and occurs in 10% to 20% of women, most often in young adulthood. These lesions are usually firm or rubbery and movable, but painless and about 1 to 3 cm in diameter. While most have single lesions, about 15% to 20% of those with fibroadenoma have multiple lesions. The character of the lesions does not change with the menstrual cycle, but lesions often enlarge during pregnancy. The lesions are comprised of monolayers of benign ductal cells with dense stroma. Fibroadenoma are usually biopsied, often by fine needle aspiration with ultrasound, to determine if they are malignant but do not require excision unless they become large or painful or the biopsy results are inconclusive. Some women may opt for excision because of concerns about the possibility of malignancy. In all cases, fibroadenoma should be monitored for changes.

Fibrocystic breast changes

The term *fibrocystic breast changes* refers to a group of nonmalignant breast lesions that are defined as follows:

- Cystic changes: these changes pertain to dilation of the ducts, which may be menses related.
- Fibrous changes: a mass may develop after an inflammatory event such as irritation of one or more ducts.
- Hyperplasia: an increase in the number of cells; this condition may have malignant potential.
- Adenosis: any change in the glandular tissue of the breast
- Papilloma: any wart-like growth in the duct system
- Ductal ectasia: refers to dilation or distention of the terminal collecting ducts

Fibrocystic breast changes are common among women older than 35 years and may be associated with caffeine intake. Physical examination may show breast nodules, most commonly in the upper outer quadrant and the axillary tail, no skin changes, and clear or white nipple discharge. The findings may change depending on menses. Nipple changes may include enlarged terminal ducts or Montgomery's glands. The differential diagnosis of any pain, mass, or changes in the breast or nipple includes carcinoma, galactorrhea, mastitis, trauma, costochondritis, adverse effects of medication, pregnancy, shingles prodrome (herpes zoster), Paget's disease, and chronic breast stimulation. Diagnostic tests may include ßHCG test, mammography, ultrasonography of the breast, and fine-needle aspiration (FNA) if the mass is palpable. Biopsy may be indicated if FNA detects bloody fluid, if the mass remains or reappears after FNA, if nipple discharge is bloody, or if there are ulcerations or scaly lesions on the nipple. Management depends on diagnosis. Decreasing caffeine intake, decreasing breast or nipple stimulation, and wearing a support brassiere may resolve the issue. If no change is noted, further testing may be indicated. If all tests indicate no suspicious masses, a trial of oral contraceptive pills may be recommended.

Hyperprolactinemia and galactorrhea

Hyperprolactinemia is an elevated serum concentration of prolactin. Galactorrhea is the secretion of milky fluid from the breast which is not related to pregnancy. Both conditions result in the secretion of a clear or milky fluid from the nipples, which may be associated with irregular menses. The findings of physical examination are usually normal; however, if a pituitary adenoma is present, funduscopic examination may show papilledema. The differential diagnosis includes pregnancy, breast cancer, thyroid disease, pituitary adenoma, excessive breast stimulation, medication side effects, ovarian disease, and brain neoplasm. Laboratory tests include TFTs, ßHCG test, serum prolactin concentration test, microscopy of secretions, and brain CT or MRI. Management depends on the cause. If the results of MRI and CT are negative, referral to an endocrinologist is warranted. If CT or MRI shows a mass, the patient should be referred to a neurosurgeon or an oncologist. If breast stimulation is the cause, then excessive manipulation should be discouraged.

Managing perimenopausal and postmenopausal vasomotor and vulvovaginal symptoms

There are several nonhormonal methods of managing perimenopausal or postmenopausal vasomotor and vulvovaginal symptoms:

- Yoga
- Meditation

- Vitamin E: some women claim some measure of relief with use, but controlled studies do not support these claims.
- Clonidine has been used but is not FDA-approved.
- Anecdotal reports suggest that soy foods and isoflavone supplements may help.

Avoiding the following may help alleviate vasomotor symptoms:

- Caffeine
- Alcohol
- Tobacco in any form
- Spicy foods
- Large meals

Regular aerobic and resistance exercise may help with problems sleeping. The following may also help with problems sleeping:

- Sleeping in a cool bedroom
- Regular sips of ice water
- Stress management
- Relaxation techniques

HRT

The indications for hormone replacement therapy (HRT) include relief of symptoms, such as hot flashes and vaginal tissue atrophy, which is related to decreased estrogen levels. Another indication is the prevention of osteoporosis. Other possible benefits may include a decreased risk of colon cancer and maintenance of memory and cognition. HRT is contraindicated if there is any history of the following:

- Thrombophlebitis or other thromboembolitic disorders
- Breast cancer
- Estrogen-dependent cancer
- Liver impairment of any type
- Uterine bleeding of undetermined cause
- Pregnancy

The following risks are associated with the use of HRT:

- Endometrial hyperplasia or cancer
- Some evidence suggests a small but significant increase in the incidence of breast cancer with long-term HRT.
- Gallbladder disease
- Disorders of the thromboembolitic system

Administration routes for HRT:

- Oral
  - o Estrogen, progestin, or combination
  - o Possible increase in HDL and triglyceride concentrations
- Transdermal patches

- o   Estrogen only or estrogen/progestin combination
- o   No evidence of elevation of HDL or triglyceride concentrations
- Vaginal estrogen creams
  - o   Help reverse postmenopausal atrophy of the vaginal lining by thickening the epithelium and increasing vaginal secretions
  - o   Also help thicken epithelium of vulvar tissue
- Estrogen vaginal ring (Estring), estradiol acetate vaginal ring (Femring)
  - o   Used to treat atrophic vaginitis due to menopause

Possible side effects of HRT are as follows:

- Breast tenderness that usually decreases after several weeks of use
- If nausea develops with oral dosage, medication should be taken at bedtime or with meals
- Transdermal patches may cause skin irritation
- Bloating may develop in some women
- Mood alteration may develop

Urinary incontinence

Urinary incontinence is defined as failure of the urinary sphincters, which causes involuntary loss of urine. Urinary incontinence can be caused by medications, nerve damage, infection, bladder neoplasms, and multiparity. Signs and symptoms include uncontrolled loss of urine when laughing, sneezing, or coughing. Physical examination may show loss of urine when an abdominal Valsalva maneuver is performed. The differential diagnosis includes UTI, bladder prolapse, vaginal atrophy, and neoplasm. Diagnostic tests include urinalysis, a voiding diary, and measurement of post-void residual. Management includes Kegel exercises to strengthen pelvic floor muscles, treatment of UTI if present, and timed-voiding exercises. A referral to a urologist is appropriate if these measures do not control the problem.

Pelvic organ prolapse

Pelvic organ prolapse occurs when pelvic floor muscles weaken with age or trauma and cannot support the pelvic organs. The uterus is the only organ that can fall into the vagina. Other organs can push against and cause a protrusion in the wall of the vagina:

- Cystocele is the bladder falling toward the vagina, causing an anterior vaginal wall protrusion.
- Urethrocele is the urethra pushing against the anterior vaginal wall, near the vaginal orifice, often occurring with a cystocele and called a cystourethrocele.
- Enterocele is part of the small intestine falling into the space between the rectum and posterior vaginal wall.
- Rectocele is the rectum protruding into the posterior vaginal wall, while a rectal prolapse is the rectum falling through the anus.
- Uterine prolapse is the uterus falling into the vagina.
- Vaginal vault prolapse is the top of the vagina falling in on itself after hysterectomy.

Pelvic organ prolapse occurs when pelvic floor muscles stretch and weaken and cannot support the pelvic organs. There are a number of different factors that contribute to this weakening:

- Trauma related to pregnancy and childbirth is the primary cause of pelvic organ prolapse because labor and birth cause stress on the pelvic muscles and ligaments, especially if forceps are used to facilitate vaginal delivery or an episiotomy is performed.
- Previous pelvic surgery, especially hysterectomy or bladder repair, may damage nerves and tissues, increasing risk for prolapse.
- Obesity exerts pressure on the pelvic floor muscles.
- Chronic cough/strain, as may occur with chronic obstructive pulmonary disease or long-term smoking, may weaken the pelvic structures over prolonged periods of time.
- Heavy lifting can cause damage to pelvic muscles.
- Spinal cord damage, whether congenital or acquired, may cause paralysis or atrophy of the pelvic muscles, thereby weakening the support.

PCO

Polycystic ovarian syndrome (PCO) is defined as a complex of symptoms including anovulation, amenorrhea, hirsutism, and obesity. The signs and symptoms of PCO are complex; however, they include a history of irregular menses, a gradual onset of hirsutism around puberty or during the early 20s, acne, male pattern baldness, a deep voice, infertility, and obesity. The differential diagnosis includes dysfunctional uterine bleeding (DUB), obesity, hyperprolactinemia, thyroid disease, Cushing's disease, and ovarian or adrenal tumors. The findings of physical examination are usually normal; however, approximately 50% of patients will have enlarged ovaries. There may be evidence of androgen excess, such as increased muscle mass, male pattern baldness, enlargement of the clitoris, and decreased breast size. Laboratory tests include a ßHCG test (to rule out pregnancy); progesterone challenge test; determination of LH, FSH, prolactin, serum testosterone, and dihydroepiandosterone sulfate (DHEAS) levels; TFTs; endometrial biopsy; and ovarian ultrasonography. Laparoscopy may be considered to determine and manage infertility.

Ovarian cysts

There are two types of ovarian cysts: functional and dermoid.

- Functional ovarian cysts occur as a result of hormonal stimulation and occur in two subcategories:
  - The follicular subcategory occurs during the follicular phase of the menstrual cycle when hormonal stimulation prevents fluid reabsorption.
  - The corpus luteum subcategory occurs during the luteal phase when the corpus luteum fails to disintegrate after ovulation.
- The dermoid type (also known as the benign cystic teratoma) is the most common ovarian germ cell tumor.

Functional or dermoid cysts can be asymptomatic or can cause severe pain if torsion or rupture occurs. If the cyst is large enough, it can cause a feeling of abdominal fullness or an aching sensation.

The physical examination may show a firm, tender, unilateral mass. Functional cysts are usually smaller than 8 cm in diameter, whereas dermoid cysts may measure 5 to 10 cm in diameter. The differential diagnosis includes pregnancy, ectopic pregnancy, ovarian torsion, fibroids, endometriosis, tubo-ovarian abscess, diverticulitis, pelvic kidney, lymphadenopathy, and neoplasm.

Diagnostic tests that should be considered include a pregnancy test, ultrasonography to evaluate the mass, and CT, MRI, or both. Management depends on the type of cyst. A functional cyst less than 6 cm in diameter in a woman of reproductive age should be examined after the next menses. Oral contraceptive pills may be considered; however, if the patient is aged 40 or older, further evaluation is suggested, and surgery may be an option. Management of a dermoid cyst includes surgical removal of the cyst and hysterectomy, salpingo-oophorectomy, or both.

Vulvar dermatosis

Vulvar dermatosis is a noncancerous disorder of the vulvar tissue. The main causes of vulvar dermatosis include lichen planus, lichen sclerosus, and lichen simplex chronicus. Lichen simplex chronicus is defined by thickening of the skin due to persistent scratching and is more common among patients with other skin conditions and chronic *Candida* infection. The physical examination may reveal skin that is easily bruised, blistered, or ulcerated; severe itching or burning; thickening or thinning of vulvar tissue; and the appearance of lesions elsewhere on the body, including the gingival and oral mucosa. The differential diagnosis includes vitiligo, carcinoma, psoriasis, *Tinea* infection, vaginitis, STD, and parasite infestation. If blisters are present, bullous pemphigoid should be considered in the differential diagnosis. Diagnostic tests may include Pap test, colposcopy, biopsy, wet mount to rule out vaginitis, KOH test of skin scrapings, and STD check. Management includes topical steroid or antifungal creams as appropriate and referral to a dermatologist.

Contraceptive practices

Cycle timing/rhythm methods

Using cycle timing/rhythm methods requires determining when the woman ovulates and abstinence from sex during the fertile phase, but pregnancy rates are about 40%, so this method is only advised if couples are very disciplined, monitor their cycles carefully, and are willing to abstain from sex for long periods during each cycle. This method is often used because of religious restrictions against artificial birth control. Ovulation detection kits (such as Ovulindex) are available OTC. They detect the enzyme guaiacol peroxidase in cervical mucosa. This indicates ovulation will occur in about six days. These kits, however, are more reliable for those attempting to become pregnant than to avoid pregnancy.

Barrier contraceptive devices

Diaphragm: This round device has a flexible supporting ring and a domelike latex cup (requiring latex allergy assessment). The concave surface (facing the cervix) is coated with spermicide before the diaphragm is inserted. The diaphragm is fitted to the individual using sized fitting rings during a pelvic exam so it seats properly below cervix and is held in place by vaginal muscles. Diaphragms range in size from 50 to 90 mm. They should not be placed more than 2 hours prior to intercourse because spermicide loses effectiveness. Diaphragms are left in place for at least 6 hours after intercourse (but not more than 12 hours). Each act of intercourse requires additional insertion of spermicide vaginally. The diaphragm should be washed with soap and water after use and inspected under bright light for tears or holes prior to each use. The diaphragm is 85% to 95% effective if used properly. Changes in weight or pregnancy can alter size requirements, so diaphragms should be refitted when either of these has occurred.

Cervical cap: This latex cap is smaller than the diaphragm (22 to 35 mm) and more cone shaped, and it fits about the cervix rather than below it. Like the diaphragm, it is used with spermicide. It may cause cervical irritation, so women may need Pap smears more frequently (every three months). It has the advantage of being able to stay in place for up to 48 hours, but leaving it in for long periods increases the risk of vaginitis and toxic shock syndrome. Cervical caps do not require additional spermicide for each act of intercourse and are 85% to 95% effective.

Female Condom: This should be used with spermicide and is 79% effective.

Contraceptive sponge: This is a donut-shaped spongy barrier device that is impregnated with nonoxynol-9 (N-9), so it is 85% to 95% effective but does not protect against STDs. The sponge has a concave central indentation on one side that fits over the cervix to act as a barrier. The outside has a string for easy removal. The sponge is left in place for 6 hours after intercourse but not more than 30 hours.

COC

Combination oral contraception (COC) is a pill taken once daily for contraception and for other selected reasons. There are two types:

- Monophasic pills deliver the same amount of active ingredient (estrogen and progestin) throughout the cycle.
- Multiphasic pills vary the amount of active ingredients throughout the cycle to more closely mimic the normal menstrual cycle.

Advantages:

- Easy to use; Can be stopped at any time
- Effective if used properly

Disadvantages:

- Does not offer protection against STDs
- Patient must be responsible enough to take pills as directed.

Contraindicated for smokers older than 35 years and for those with a history of any of the following:

- Deep vein thrombosis (DVT); Pulmonary embolus; Stroke. Ischemic heart disease; Pulmonary hypertension. Subacute bacterial endocarditis (SBE). Nephropathy, retinopathy, or neuropathy due to diabetes; Diabetes for 20 years or more; Pregnancy; Breast cancer; Migraine headaches

Depo-Provera

Medroxyprogesterone acetate (Depo-Provera) is an injectable contraceptive that prevents ovulation. It is given as an intramuscular injection in the upper arm or buttock every three months.

Advantages:

- Ease of use: the injection is needed only every three months
- Reversible: patient can stop injections at any time
- After approximately one year of use, amenorrhea can occur; it is reversible once injections are stopped.
- Effective in preventing pregnancy
- Can be used by a woman who is breastfeeding

Disadvantages

- Irregular and unpredictable bleeding can occur
- Weight gain; Headaches;
- Does not prevent the transmission of STDs
- Calcium loss: women using this medication should take a calcium supplement and should participate in resistance training to mobilize calcium deposition into the bones.

Contraindicated for women with a history of any of the following: Liver disease; Deep vein thrombosis (DVT); Occult vaginal bleeding; Pregnancy; Breast cancer; Any cancer of the reproductive system

Norplant

The progestin-only implant (Norplant) is a five-year birth control method that consists of six short silicone rods impregnated with progestin which are implanted under the skin in the upper arm.

Advantages:

- Ease of use
- Effective in preventing pregnancy
- Fertility returns once rods are removed
- Can be used during breastfeeding
- Long-term contraception

Disadvantages:

- Irregular and unpredictable bleeding
- Headaches; Acne; Weight gain
- Nausea; No protection against STDs
- Minor surgical procedure needed for insertion; however, removal may be difficult.

Contraindicated for women with a history of any of the following:

- Liver disease; Breast cancer
- Deep vein thrombosis (DVT); Stroke
- Migraine headaches; Occult vaginal bleeding

Note: The distribution of Norplant was stopped in the United States in 2002, but Norplant was still available until 2004; therefore, nurse practitioners and other clinicians may still see patients with Norplant inserts.

Transdermal contraceptive system

The transdermal contraceptive system (TCS) is a patch that is applied to the skin and delivers a controlled dose of progestin and estrogen. The patient replaces the patch each week for three weeks and wears no patch for one week; the absence of the patch for this week will cause menstruation.

Advantages:

- Easy to use; no need to remember to take pills
- Can be stopped at any time
- Highly effective
- Patient has control of her menstrual cycle.

Disadvantages:

- Does not offer protection against STDs
- Skin at the application site can become irritated.

Contraindicated for smokers older than 35 years and for those with a history of any of the following:

- Deep vein thrombosis (DVT); Pulmonary embolus
- Stroke; Ischemic heart disease; Pulmonary hypertension
- Subacute bacterial endocarditis (SBE)
- Nephropathy, retinopathy, or neuropathy due to diabetes
- Diabetes for 20 years or more; Pregnancy; Breast cancer
- Migraine headaches

NuvaRing

The Contraceptive Vaginal Ring (NuvaRing) is a soft plastic ring worn in the vagina for three weeks; the ring is not worn for one week to allow menses. The ring delivers a dose of estrogen and progestin.

Advantages:

- Easy to use. Effect is reversible.
- Effective in preventing pregnancy. Patient has control of her menstrual cycle.

Disadvantages:

- Does not prevent the transmission of STDs
- Patient must be responsible enough to change ring weekly.
- Vaginal irritation or discharge

Contraindicated for smokers older than 35 years and for those with a history of any of the following:

- Deep vein thrombosis (DVT)
- Pulmonary embolus; Stroke
- Ischemic heart disease
- Pulmonary hypertension
- Subacute bacterial endocarditis (SBE)
- Nephropathy, retinopathy, or neuropathy due to diabetes
- Diabetes for 20 years or more
- Pregnancy; Breast cancer; Migraine headaches

Vaginal spermicides

Vaginal spermicides are medications that destroy sperm. These medications, which are placed into the vagina, come in a variety of forms: foams, creams, suppositories, tablets, and gel.

Mechanism of action:

- Active ingredient is usually Octoxynol-9 or Nonoxynol-9.
- Destroys the cell membrane of the sperm

Advantages:

- Easy accessibility
- Inexpensive
- Can be used as a back-up birth control option
- No systemic effects

Disadvantages:

- No protection against STDs
- Can be messy to use
- Possible reactions, such as skin irritation, for both woman and man

Special instructions:

- Contraception will be more effective if spermicide is used with another contraceptive method, such as a condom, cervical cap, or diaphragm.
- If spermicide is inserted too soon before vaginal intercourse, pregnancy may result.
- Place spermicide deep in the vagina.

Emergency contraception

Emergency contraception (the morning-after pill) is used to prevent unintended contraception after unprotected vaginal intercourse.

Mechanism of actions:

- Interferes with ovulation
- Interferes with transport of sperm and ova

Advantages

- Provides contraception in the event of:
  - o Unplanned vaginal intercourse
  - o Failure of intended contraceptive method:
    - ❖ Condom breakage or leakage
    - ❖ Cervical cap improperly placed or dislodged
    - ❖ Missed birth control pills
    - ❖ Missed or late contraceptive injection
  - o Rape

Disadvantages:

- Nausea; Vomiting; Menstrual irregularities

Contraindication:

- Positive results of urine pregnancy test or βHCG test

Medication used

- Levonorgestrel (Plan B): Two 0.75-mg doses given 12 hours apart
  - Must be used within 72 hours of unprotected sex
  - Promethazine (Phenergan): 25 mg BID if nausea or vomiting develops

Permanent female sterilization

Permanent female sterilization is a surgical procedure that results in permanent contraception.

Mechanism of action:

- The patient's fallopian tubes are obstructed to prevent sperm from uniting with the egg.

Two methods:

- The tube is cut, and the clipped ends are cauterized, clipped, or both.
- The tube is only clipped.

Advantages:

- Permanent sterilization
- Long-term cost-effectiveness
- Because pregnancy is no longer a concern, sex life may improve.

Disadvantages:

- Surgical procedure that requires general anesthesia
- Should be considered nonreversible
- Does not protect against STDs
- Initial expense is high

Contraception for women aged 40 or older

Contraception should be continued until the patient has had no periods for one full year. The following are birth control options:

- Low-dose oral contraceptives
  - Noncontraceptive benefits such as a decreased incidence of endometrial and ovarian cancer and minimization of hot flashes may be especially appealing to the perimenopausal woman.
- Intrauterine device (IUD)
  - Long-lasting contraceptive system with no concern about taking pills and missing doses

- o IUD impregnated with levonorgestrel may also help control the heavy bleeding that some perimenopausal women experience.
- Barrier devices, such as the cervical cap, should be discussed.
- Permanent sterilization (tubal ligation) is the most common form of birth control among married women in the United States.

Induced abortion

Induced abortion may be done before the time of fetal viability (up to 24 weeks), but increasingly state regulations are limiting access to late-term abortions.

Surgical procedures

Surgical procedure	Gestation	Discussion
Vacuum aspiration	4 to 10 weeks	This may be done manually or by machine, with a cervical dilator used first and then a cannula passed into the uterus to suction the tissue
Suction curettage	6 to 14 weeks	This is similar to vacuum aspiration, but a looped curettage is inserted into the uterus after the tissue is suctioned to remove any remnants.
Dilation and extraction	14 to 24 weeks	The cervix is dilated, and the fetus extracted by instrument, usually followed by suctioning to remove remnants. This procedure is common during the second trimester.
Intact dilation and extraction	> 18 weeks	This "partial birth abortion" usually follows induced labor and removes the intact fetus via the cervix, but it requires prior feticide (intra-amniotic or interfetal digoxin or potassium chloride) to prevent live birth.
Hysterectomy/ hysterotomy	12 to 24 weeks	This procedure is used only as a last resort (rare).

Medical procedures

Medical procedures for induced abortion can be used during the first trimester. Because medication-induced abortion always involves cramping and heavy bleeding, supervision should be available in case hemorrhage occurs.

Medications	Discussion
Mifepristone-misoprostol	Mifepristone is administered orally on day 1 to block action of progesterone and change endometrium and then misoprostol vaginally or buccally on day 2 or 3 (or within 8 hours if bleeding is occurring) to cause contractions to help expel the embryo/fetus. Medical examination to ensure abortion complete is done after 7 days.
Methotrexate-misoprostol	Methotrexate injection is administered on day 1 to stop cell division and growth of the embryo followed by misoprostol vaginally on day 6 or 7 with examination on day 8 to ensure that abortion is complete.

In some cases, misoprostol or mifepristone may be used alone. If abortion is incomplete after medication-induced abortion, then suction and curettage may be necessary to remove retained tissue.

Adoption

A mother relinquishing her child for adoption may have feelings of ambivalence and sadness. Many who relinquish their infants for adoption are young and/or unmarried. Adoptions may be closed or open, so procedures will vary. In some open adoptions, the adoptive parent(s) may accompany the mother and participate in the birth, with the birth mother relinquishing the child immediately after birth. In this case, the adoptive parents should be treated as the actual parents of the child while still recognizing the needs of the birth mother and providing her emotional and physical support. In other cases, the child is first relinquished to an agency, such as social services, which then places the child. If possible, prior to the birth, the birth mother should indicate how she wants to handle the birth. Some want to hold and spend time with the child; others do not. The birth mother should be in a single room rather than with other mothers to protect her privacy.

Options counseling

Options counseling provides the pregnant woman and sometimes her partner with information about legal and medical options related to her pregnancy and nonjudgmental support. Most women seek options counseling because of stress, fear regarding pregnancy, or unwanted pregnancy and may want help in making a decision about terminating or continuing the pregnancy. The counselor should avoid trying to influence the woman's decision but should remain empathetic and provide complete information. Discussion should include:

- Childbirth: Different types of delivery choices, financial support, community support, and available welfare assistance. Females may need strategies to inform parents or partners.
- Abortion: Both surgical and medical options, including description of procedures, complications, and limitations related to weeks of gestation.
- Adoption: Various options, including private (arranged by an attorney or private adoption agency) or public (arranged through governmental adoption services). Open versus closed adoptions should be explored.

Male sexual dysfunction

Erectile dysfunction (ED—impotence)
- Inability to achieve or maintain an adequate erection for intercourse
- ED may relate to psychological (anxiety, depression, fatigue), environmental (smoking, alcohol use) or organic factors (occlusive vascular disease); diabetes; pituitary tumors; thyroid dysfunction; testosterone deficiency; or chronic renal failure. Obesity may also contribute to ED. Prostatectomy or other surgery may result in ED.
- Medications that may cause erectile dysfunction include antihypertensives, antiadrenergics, anticholinergics, phenothiazines, anticonvulsants, antifungals, antihormones, antipsychotics, SSRIs, anxiolytics, beta blockers, calcium channel blockers, carbonic anhydrate inhibitors, H2 antagonists, NSAIDs, thiazide diuretics, and tricyclic antidepressants.

Treatment includes oral medications (Viagra, Cialis), testosterone, external vacuum tumescence devices (an elastic ring at the base of the penis inhibits venous drainage to maintain erection), intracorporeal (injection into corpus cavernosa) or intraurethral (small pellet inserted with an applicator) medications, and penile prosthesis (surgical procedure if other means fail).

Premature ejaculation

Lack of voluntary control over ejaculation results in ejaculation occurring before penetration or shortly after. While this may occur in all men at times, if it happens routinely, the man should practice relaxation to reduce anxiety as well as other techniques with a partner to prolong time to ejaculation:

- Stop/start: Stimulate until almost the point of orgasm, stop, wait 30 seconds, and start again, repeating until the man chooses to complete ejaculation.
- Squeeze: Stimulate until almost the point of orgasm, stop, squeeze the end of the penis for a few seconds until the urge passes, wait 30 seconds, start again, repeating the cycle until the man chooses to complete ejaculation.

SSRIs, which tend to prolong time to ejaculation, may be helpful if other methods fail. Condoms or local anesthetic cream applied to the end of the penis may reduce sensation and stimulation, delaying ejaculation.

Male contraceptive practices

Vasectomy

The male's vas deferens are clipped or severed and then tied or sealed under local anesthetic. The procedure is done with one central puncture or bilateral incisions. Other birth control methods must be used for 4 to 6 weeks. It may take up to 36 ejaculations to clear the remaining sperm. A sperm count is done at 6 weeks with follow-up at 6 and 12 months to check for recanalization that might restore fertility. Discomfort is usually minimal. Complications include infection, pain, hematoma, and recurrent epididymitis. Reversal techniques are 30% to 85% effective.

Male condom

These are more effective if used with spermicide, but nonoxynol-9 (N-9) should be avoided because it interferes with protection against sexually transmitted diseases. Patients should have instruction in proper use to avoid semen leaking from the male condom. Male condoms are 80% to 90% effective.

Coitus interruptus

Coitus interruptus, also known as the "withdrawal" method, is a contraceptive method that requires the male to withdraw his penis from the vagina before ejaculation.

Mechanism of action:

- No contact between egg and sperm

Advantages:

- No medications involved
- No monetary expense

Disadvantages:

- Male partner must exercise self-control
- Not recommended if premature ejaculation is an issue
- Does not protect against STDs

- Caution: If any semen is deposited on the external female genitalia, there is the slim chance that sperm can enter the vagina and survive long enough to fertilize an egg.
- If several acts of coitus occur, sperm from previous sex acts may lie in the urethra. These sperm can enter the vagina during subsequent sexual intercourse, resulting in the possibility of pregnancy.

Male sexually transmitted infection

Human papillomavirus

Human papillomavirus (HPV) includes > 40 that are sexually transmitted and invade mucosal tissue, causing genital warts (condylomata). HPV infection causes changes in the mucosa, which can lead to penile cancer in males and cervical cancer in females. Over 99% of cervical cancers are caused by HPV. Most HPVs cause little or no overt symptoms in males or females. Men are at risk for development of both HPV-related penile as well as anal cancer (usually related to men having sex with other men). HPV can also be spread to the mouth and throat of a partner engaging in oral sex with an infected person, leading to head and neck cancer. Signs of genital warts include wartlike raised or flat lesions about the external genitalia. Lesions may occur within a few weeks or months after sexual contact. Indications of penile cancer include change in the color of the skin on the penis and thickening initially with a painless sore appearing in later stages. The HPV vaccine Gardasil should be given before initial sexual contact.

Chlamydia

Most males are asymptomatic, but symptoms may occur ≤ 3 weeks after exposure and can include inflammation of the mouth or throat, proctitis, burning urination, and conjunctivitis. Severe infection may cause fever, night sweats, prostatitis, painful ejaculation, hematuria, low back pain, and erectile dysfunction. Treatment is antibiotics.

Gonorrhea

Many males are asymptomatic. Those with symptoms may have penile pain, lower abdominal discomfort, purulent discharge (white to yellow to green), and burning on urination. Some also develop a sore mouth or throat and eye inflammation and discharge. Treatment is antibiotics.

Syphilis

Stage I: A painless chancre develops on the penis or site of infection (mouth, anus) 10 to 90 days after infection. Syphilis spreads easily to the female in this stage. Treatment with antibiotics is necessary to prevent progress to stages II and III.

Trichomonas

Most males are asymptomatic or have only mild symptoms, such as penile irritation and slight burning on urination or ejaculation.

Important terms

- Menopause - The time when menses ends; authenticated after 12 consecutive months pass without a period
- Climacteric/perimenopause - Interchangeable terms used for the transition from the reproductive to the nonreproductive condition. This transition period is marked by decreased production of estrogen and progesterone. Irregular periods, another hallmark of the climacteric/perimenopausal phase, occur because the decrease in the number of active follicles causes decreased production of estradiol. At the end of the climacteric (the beginning of menopause), the ovaries contain no follicles; thus, the endometrium atrophies. Fertility ends at this time.
- Postmenopause - The period of life that follows menopause. FSH and LH levels are elevated.
- Premature menopause - The occurrence of menopause before the woman reaches the age of 40 years